Skill Checklists for

Fundamentals of Nursing

THE ART AND SCIENCE OF PERSON-CENTERED
NURSING CARE

Skill Checklists for

Fundamentals of Nursing

THE ART AND SCIENCE OF PERSON-CENTERED NURSING CARE

EIGHTH EDITION

Carol Taylor, PhD, MSN, RN
Professor of Nursing
Georgetown University School of Nursing and Health Studies
Washington, DC

Carol Lillis, MSN, RN
Faculty Emerita
Delaware County Community College
Media, Pennsylvania

Pamela Lynn, MSN, RN
Instructor
Gwynedd Mercy University
Frances M. Maguire School of Nursing and Health Professions
Gwynedd Valley, Pennsylvania

. Wolters Kluwer

Philadelphia · Baltimore · New York · London
Buenos Aires · Hong Kong · Sydney · Tokyo

Publisher: Lisa McAllister
Executive Editor: Sherry Dickinson
Product Development Editor: Helen Kogut
Editorial Assistant: Dan Reilly
Marketing Manager: Dean Karampelas
Production Project Manager: Cynthia Rudy
Design Coordinator: Holly Reid McLaughlin
Illustration Coordinator: Jennifer Clements
Manufacturing Coordinator: Karin Duffield
Prepress Vendor: Aptara, Inc.

8th Edition

Introduction

Developing clinical competency is an important challenge for each fundamentals nursing student. To facilitate the mastery of nursing skills, we are happy to provide skill checklists for each skill included in *Fundamentals of Nursing: The Art and Science of Person-Centered Nursing Care*, Eighth Edition. Students can use the checklists to facilitate self-evaluation, and faculty will find them useful in measuring and recording student performance. Three-hole-punched and perforated, these checklists can be easily reproduced and brought to the simulation laboratory or clinical area.

The checklists follow each step of the skill to provide a complete evaluative tool. They are designed to record an evaluation of each step of the procedure.

- Checkmark in the "Excellent" column denotes mastering the procedure.
- Checkmark in the "Satisfactory" column indicates use of the recommended technique.
- Checkmark in the "Needs Practice" column indicates use of some but not all of each recommended technique.

The Comments section allows you to highlight suggestions that will improve skills. Space is available at the top of each checklist to record a final pass/fail evaluation, date, and the signature of the student and evaluating faculty member.

Faculty who adopt this book will also find on thePoint website at http://thepoint.lww.com/TaylorCklst8e a *Master Skills Competency Checklist* to aid in record keeping.

List of Skills by Chapter

List of Skills in Alphabetical Order

Skill Checklists for Fundamentals of Nursing:
The Art and Science of Person-Centered Nursing Care, 8th edition

Name _____   Date _____

Unit _____   Position _____

Instructor/Evaluator: _____   Position _____

SKILL 23-1
Performing Hand Hygiene Using Soap and Water (Handwashing)

Goal: The hands will be free of visible soiling and transient microorganisms will be eliminated.

Excellent	Satisfactory	Needs Practice		Comments
____	____	____	1. Gather the necessary supplies. Stand in front of the sink. Do not allow your clothing to touch the sink during the washing procedure.	
____	____	____	2. Remove jewelry, if possible, and secure in a safe place. A plain wedding band may remain in place.	
____	____	____	3. Turn on water and adjust force. Regulate the temperature until the water is warm.	
____	____	____	4. Wet the hands and wrist area. Keep hands lower than elbows to allow water to flow toward fingertips.	
____	____	____	5. Use about 1 teaspoon liquid soap from dispenser or rinse bar of soap and lather thoroughly. Cover all areas of hands with the soap product. Rinse soap bar again and return to soap rack without touching the rack.	
____	____	____	6. With firm rubbing and circular motions, wash the palms and backs of the hands, each finger, the areas between the fingers, and the knuckles, wrists, and forearms. *Wash at least 1 inch above area of contamination.* If hands are not visibly soiled, wash to 1 inch above the wrists.	
____	____	____	7. Continue this friction motion for at least 20 seconds.	
____	____	____	8. Use fingernails of the opposite hand or a clean orangewood stick to clean under fingernails.	
____	____	____	9. Rinse thoroughly with water flowing toward fingertips.	
____	____	____	10. Pat hands dry with a paper towel, beginning with the fingers and moving upward toward forearms, and discard it immediately. Use another clean towel to turn off the faucet. Discard towel immediately without touching other clean hand.	
____	____	____	11. Use oil-free lotion on hands if desired.	

Skill Checklists for Fundamentals of Nursing:
The Art and Science of Person-Centered Nursing Care, 8th edition

Name _____   Date _____

Unit _____   Position _____

Instructor/Evaluator: _____   Position _____

Excellent	Satisfactory	Needs Practice	SKILL 23-2 **Using Personal Protective Equipment (PPE)**	
			Goal: The transmission of microorganisms is prevented.	**Comments**
——	——	——	1. Check medical record and nursing plan of care for type of precautions and review precautions in infection control manual.	
——	——	——	2. Plan nursing activities before entering patient's room.	
——	——	——	3. Perform hand hygiene.	
——	——	——	4. Provide instruction about precautions to patient, family members, and visitors.	
——	——	——	5. Put on gown, mask, protective eyewear, and gloves based on the type of exposure anticipated and category of isolation precautions.	
——	——	——	a. Put on the gown, with the opening in the back. Tie gown securely at neck and waist.	
——	——	——	b. Put on the mask or respirator over your nose, mouth, and chin. Secure ties or elastic bands at the middle of the head and neck. If respirator is used, perform a fit check. Inhale; the respirator should collapse. Exhale; air should not leak out.	
——	——	——	c. Put on goggles. Place over eyes and adjust to fit. Alternately, a face shield could be used to take the place of the mask and goggles.	
——	——	——	d. Put on clean disposable gloves. Extend gloves to cover the cuffs of the gown.	
——	——	——	6. Identify the patient. Explain the procedure to the patient. Continue with patient care as appropriate.	
			Remove PPE	
——	——	——	7. Remove PPE: Except for respirator, remove PPE at the doorway or in an anteroom. *Remove respirator after leaving the patient's room and closing the door.*	
——	——	——	a. If impervious gown has been tied in front of the body at the waistline, untie waist strings before removing gloves.	
——	——	——	b. Grasp the outside of one glove with the opposite gloved hand and peel off, turning the glove inside out as you pull it off. Hold the removed glove in the remaining gloved hand.	

Using Personal Protective Equipment (PPE) *(Continued)*

Excellent **Satisfactory** **Needs Practice**

Comments

____ ____ ____   c. Slide fingers of ungloved hand under the remaining glove at the wrist, *taking care not to touch the outer surface of the glove.*

____ ____ ____   d. Peel off the glove over the first glove, containing the one glove inside the other. Discard in appropriate container.

____ ____ ____   e. To remove the goggles or face shield: Handle by the headband or earpieces. Lift away from the face. Place in designated receptacle for reprocessing or in an appropriate waste container.

____ ____ ____   f. To remove gown: Unfasten ties, if at the neck and back. Allow the gown to fall away from shoulders. *Touching only the inside of the gown,* pull away from the torso. Keeping hands on the inner surface of the gown, pull gown from arms. Turn gown inside out. Fold or roll into a bundle and discard.

____ ____ ____   g. To remove mask or respirator: Grasp the neck ties or elastic, then top ties or elastic and remove. *Take care to avoid touching front of mask or respirator.* Discard in waste container. If using a respirator, save for future use in the designated area.

____ ____ ____ 8. Perform hand hygiene immediately after removing all PPE.

Skill Checklists for Fundamentals of Nursing:
The Art and Science of Person-Centered Nursing Care, 8th edition

Name _____ Date _____

Unit _____ Position _____

Instructor/Evaluator: _____ Position _____

SKILL 23-3

Preparing a Sterile Field and Adding Sterile Items to a Sterile Field

Goal: The sterile field is created without contamination and the patient remains free of exposure to potential infection-causing microorganisms.

Excellent	Satisfactory	Needs Practice		Comments
___	___	___	1. Perform hand hygiene and put on PPE, if indicated.	
___	___	___	2. Identify the patient. Explain the procedure to the patient.	
			Preparing a Sterile Field	
___	___	___	3. Check that packaged sterile drape is dry and unopened. Also, note expiration date, making sure that the date is still valid.	
___	___	___	4. Select a work area that is waist level or higher.	
___	___	___	5. Open sterile wrapped drape or commercially prepared kit following the directions below.	
			For a Prepackaged Sterile Drape	
___	___	___	a. Open the outer covering of the drape. Remove sterile drape, lifting it carefully by its corners. Hold away from body and above the waist and work surface.	
___	___	___	b. Continue to hold only by the corners. Allow the drape to unfold, away from your body and any other surface.	
___	___	___	c. Position the drape on the work surface with the moisture-proof side down. This would be the shiny or blue side. Avoid touching any other surface or object with the drape. If any portion of the drape hangs off the work surface, that part of the drape is considered contaminated. Do not touch or reach over the sterile field.	
			For a Commercially Prepared Kit or Tray	
___	___	___	a. Open the outside cover of the package and remove the kit or tray. Place in the center of the work surface, with the topmost flap positioned on the far side of the package. Discard outside cover.	
___	___	___	b. Reach around the package and grasp the outer surface of the end of the topmost flap, holding no more than 1 inch from the border of the flap. Pull open away from the body, keeping the arm outstretched and away from the inside of the wrapper. Allow the wrapper to lie flat on the work surface.	

Preparing a Sterile Field and Adding
Sterile Items to a Sterile Field *(Continued)*

Excellent	Satisfactory	Needs Practice		Comments

c. Reach around the package and grasp the outer surface of the first side flap, holding no more than 1 inch from the border of the flap. Pull open to the side of the package, keeping the arm outstretched and away from the inside of the wrapper. Allow the wrapper to lie flat on the work surface.

d. Reach around the package and grasp the outer surface of the remaining side flap, holding no more than 1 inch from the border of the flap. Pull open to the side of the package, keeping the arm outstretched and away from the inside of the wrapper. Allow the wrapper to lie flat on the work surface.

e. Stand away from the package and work surface. Grasp the outer surface of the remaining flap closest to the body, holding not more than 1 inch from the border of the flap. Pull the flap back toward the body, keeping arm outstretched and away from the inside of the wrapper. Keep this hand in place. Use other hand to grasp the wrapper on the underside (the side that is down to the work surface). Position the wrapper so that when flat, edges are on the work surface, and do not hang down over sides of work surface. Allow the wrapper to lie flat on the work surface.

f. The outer wrapper of the package has become a sterile field with the packaged supplies in the center. Do not touch or reach over the sterile field.

Adding Items to a Sterile Field

6. Place additional sterile items on field as needed.

To Add an Agency-Wrapped and Sterilized Item

a. Hold agency-wrapped item in the dominant hand, with top flap opening away from the body. With other hand, reach around the package and unfold top flap and both sides.

b. Keep a secure hold on item through the wrapper with the dominant hand. Grasp the remaining flap of the wrapper closest to the body, taking care not to touch the inner surface of the wrapper or the item. Pull the flap back toward the wrist, so the wrapper covers the hand and wrist.

Preparing a Sterile Field and Adding Sterile Items to a Sterile Field *(Continued)*

Excellent	Satisfactory	Needs Practice		Comments

c. Grasp all the corners of the wrapper together with the nondominant hand and pull back toward wrist, covering hand and wrist. Hold in place.

d. Hold the item 6 inches above the surface of the sterile field and drop onto the field. Be careful to avoid touching the surface or other items or dropping onto the 1-inch border.

To Add a Commercially Wrapped and Sterilized Item

a. Hold package in one hand. Pull back top cover with other hand. Alternately, carefully peel the edges apart using both hands.

b. After top cover or edges are partially separated, hold the item 6 inches above the surface of the sterile field. Continue opening the package and drop the item onto the field. *Be careful to avoid touching the surface or other items or dropping onto the 1-inch border.*

c. Discard wrapper.

To Add a Sterile Solution

a. Obtain appropriate solution and check expiration date.

b. Open solution container according to directions and *place cap on table away from the field with edges up.*

c. Hold bottle outside the edge of the sterile field with the label side facing the palm of your hand and prepare to pour from a height of 4 to 6 inches (10 to 15 cm). *Never touch the tip of the bottle to the sterile container or field.*

d. Pour required amount of solution steadily into sterile container previously added to sterile field and positioned at side of sterile field or onto dressings. *Avoid splashing any liquid.*

e. Touch only the outside of the lid when recapping. Label solution with date and time of opening.

7. Continue with the procedure as indicated.

8. When procedure is completed, remove PPE, if used. Perform hand hygiene.

Skill Checklists for Fundamentals of Nursing:
The Art and Science of Person-Centered Nursing Care, 8th edition

Name _____   Date _____

Unit _____   Position _____

Instructor/Evaluator: _____   Position _____

SKILL 23-4

Putting on Sterile Gloves and Removing Soiled Gloves

Goal: The gloves are applied and removed without contamination.

Excellent	Satisfactory	Needs Practice		Comments
——	——	——	1. Perform hand hygiene and put on PPE, if indicated.	
——	——	——	2. Identify the patient. Explain the procedure to the patient.	
——	——	——	3. Check that the sterile glove package is dry and unopened. Also note expiration date, making sure that the date is still valid.	
——	——	——	4. Place sterile glove package on clean, dry surface at or above your waist.	
——	——	——	5. Open the outside wrapper by carefully peeling the top layer back. Remove inner package, handling only the outside of it.	
——	——	——	6. Place the inner package on the work surface with the side labeled "cuff end" closest to the body.	
——	——	——	7. Carefully open the inner package. Fold open the top flap, then the bottom and sides. *Take care not to touch the inner surface of the package or the gloves.*	
——	——	——	8. With the thumb and forefinger of the nondominant hand, grasp the folded cuff of the glove for the dominant hand, touching only the exposed inside of the glove.	
——	——	——	9. Keeping the hands above the waistline, lift and hold the glove up and off the inner package with fingers down. *Be careful that it does not touch any unsterile object.*	
——	——	——	10. Carefully insert dominant hand palm up into glove and pull glove on. Leave the cuff folded until the opposite hand is gloved.	
——	——	——	11. Hold the thumb of the gloved hand outward. Place the fingers of the gloved hand inside the cuff of the remaining glove. Lift it from the wrapper, taking care not to touch anything with the gloves or hands.	
——	——	——	12. Carefully insert nondominant hand into glove. Pull the glove on, taking care that the skin does not touch any of the outer surfaces of the gloves.	

Excellent	Satisfactory	Needs Practice		Comments
			SKILL 23-4 **Putting on Sterile Gloves and Removing Soiled Gloves** *(Continued)*	

Excellent	Satisfactory	Needs Practice		Comments
—	—	—	13. *Slide the fingers of one hand under the cuff of the other and fully extend the cuff down the arm, touching only the sterile outside of the glove. Repeat for the remaining hand.*	
—	—	—	14. Adjust gloves on both hands if necessary, *touching only sterile areas with other sterile areas.*	
—	—	—	15. Continue with procedure as indicated.	
			Removing Soiled Gloves	
—	—	—	16. Use dominant hand to grasp the opposite glove *near cuff end on the outside exposed area.* Remove it by pulling it off, inverting it as it is pulled, keeping the contaminated area on the inside. Hold the removed glove in the remaining gloved hand.	
—	—	—	17. Slide fingers of ungloved hand between the remaining glove and the wrist. *Take care to avoid touching the outside surface of the glove.* Remove it by pulling it off, inverting it as it is pulled, keeping the contaminated area on the inside, and securing the first glove inside the second.	
—	—	—	18. Discard gloves in appropriate container. Remove additional PPE, if used. Perform hand hygiene.	

Skill Checklists for Fundamentals of Nursing:
The Art and Science of Person-Centered Nursing Care, 8th edition

Name _____ Date _____

Unit _____ Position _____

Instructor/Evaluator: _____ Position _____

Excellent	**Satisfactory**	**Needs Practice**	

SKILL 24-1

Assessing Body Temperature

Goal: The patient's temperature is assessed accurately without injury and the patient experiences only minimal discomfort. **Comments**

Excellent	Satisfactory	Needs Practice		Comments
——	——	——	1. Check the medical order or nursing care plan for frequency of measurement and route. More frequent temperature measurement may be appropriate based on nursing judgment.	
——	——	——	2. Perform hand hygiene and put on PPE, if indicated.	
——	——	——	3. Identify the patient.	
——	——	——	4. Close the curtains around the bed and close the door to the room, if possible. Discuss the procedure with the patient and assess the patient's ability to assist with the procedure.	
——	——	——	5. Assemble equipment on the overbed table within reach.	
——	——	——	6. Ensure that the electronic or digital thermometer is in working condition.	
——	——	——	7. Put on gloves, if indicated.	
——	——	——	8. Select the appropriate site based on previous assessment data.	
——	——	——	9. Follow the steps as outlined below for the appropriate type of thermometer.	
——	——	——	10. When measurement is completed, remove gloves, if worn. Remove additional PPE, if used. Perform hand hygiene.	

Measuring an Oral Temperature

Excellent	Satisfactory	Needs Practice		Comments
——	——	——	11. Remove the electronic unit from the charging unit, and remove the probe from within the recording unit.	
——	——	——	12. Cover thermometer probe with disposable probe cover and slide it on until it snaps into place.	
——	——	——	13. *Place the probe beneath the patient's tongue in the posterior sublingual pocket. Ask the patient to close his or her lips around the probe.*	
——	——	——	14. Continue to hold the probe until you hear a beep. Note the temperature reading.	
——	——	——	15. Remove the probe from the patient's mouth. Dispose of the probe cover by holding the probe over an appropriate receptacle and pressing the probe release button.	

Excellent	Satisfactory	Needs Practice		Comments

SKILL 24-1
Assessing Body Temperature *(Continued)*

——— ——— ——— 16. Return the thermometer probe to the storage place within the unit. Return the electronic unit to the charging unit, if appropriate.

Measuring a Tympanic Membrane Temperature

——— ——— ——— 17. If necessary, push the "ON" button and wait for the "ready" signal on the unit.

——— ——— ——— 18. Slide the disposable cover onto the tympanic probe.

——— ——— ——— 19. *Insert the probe snugly into the external ear using gentle but firm pressure, angling the thermometer toward the patient's jaw line. Pull the pinna up and back to straighten the ear canal in an adult.*

——— ——— ——— 20. Activate the unit by pushing the trigger button. The reading is immediate (usually within 2 seconds). Note the reading.

——— ——— ——— 21. Discard the probe cover in an appropriate receptacle by pushing the probe-release button or use the rim of cover to remove it from the probe. Replace the thermometer in its charger, if necessary.

Measuring Temporal Artery Temperature

——— ——— ——— 22. Brush the patient's hair aside if it is covering the temporal artery area.

——— ——— ——— 23. Apply a probe cover.

——— ——— ——— 24. Hold the thermometer like a remote control device, with your thumb on the red "ON" button. Place the probe flush on the center of the forehead, with the body of the instrument sideways (not straight up and down), so that it is not in the patient's face.

——— ——— ——— 25. Depress the "ON" button. Keep the button depressed throughout the measurement.

——— ——— ——— 26. Slowly slide the probe straight across the forehead, midline, to the hairline. The thermometer will click; fast clicking indicates a rise to a higher temperature, slow clicking indicates that the instrument is still scanning, but not finding any higher temperature.

——— ——— ——— 27. Brush hair aside if it is covering the ear, exposing the area of the neck under the ear lobe. Lift the probe from the forehead and touch on the neck just behind the ear lobe, in the depression just below the mastoid.

——— ——— ——— 28. Release the button and read the thermometer measurement.

Excellent	Satisfactory	Needs Practice	SKILL 24-1 **Assessing Body Temperature** *(Continued)*	Comments
——	——	——	29. Hold the thermometer over a waste receptacle. Gently push the probe cover with your thumb against the proximal edge to dispose of the probe cover.	
——	——	——	30. The instrument will automatically turn off in 30 seconds, or press and release the power button.	
			Measuring Axillary Temperature	
——	——	——	31. Move the patient's clothing to expose only the axilla.	
——	——	——	32. Remove the probe from the recording unit of the electronic thermometer. Place a disposable probe cover on by sliding it on and snapping it securely.	
——	——	——	33. *Place the end of the probe in the center of the axilla. Have the patient bring the arm down and close to the body.*	
——	——	——	34. Hold the probe in place until you hear a beep, and then carefully remove the probe. Note the temperature reading.	
——	——	——	35. Cover the patient and help the patient to a position of comfort.	
——	——	——	36. Dispose of the probe cover by holding the probe over an appropriate waste receptacle and pushing the release button.	
——	——	——	37. Place the bed in the lowest position and elevate rails, as needed. Leave the patient clean and comfortable.	
——	——	——	38. Return the electronic thermometer to the charging unit.	
			Measuring Rectal Temperature	
——	——	——	39. Adjust the bed to a comfortable working height, usually elbow height of the care giver (VISN 8 Patient Safety Center, 2012). Put on nonsterile gloves.	
——	——	——	40. Assist the patient to a side-lying position. Pull back the covers sufficiently to expose only the buttocks.	
——	——	——	41. Remove the rectal probe from within the recording unit of the electronic thermometer. Cover the probe with a disposable probe cover and slide it into place until it snaps in place.	
——	——	——	42. *Lubricate about 1 inch of the probe with a water-soluble lubricant.*	
——	——	——	43. Reassure the patient. Separate the buttocks until the anal sphincter is clearly visible.	
——	——	——	44. *Insert the thermometer probe into the anus about 1.5 inches in an adult or no more than 1 inch in a child.*	

SKILL 24-1

Assessing Body Temperature *(Continued)*

Excellent	Satisfactory	Needs Practice		Comments
——	——	——	45. Hold the probe in place until you hear a beep, then carefully remove the probe. Note the temperature reading on the display.	
——	——	——	46. Dispose of the probe cover by holding the probe over an appropriate waste receptacle and pressing the release button.	
——	——	——	47. Using toilet tissue, wipe the anus of any feces or excess lubricant. Dispose of the toilet tissue. Remove gloves and discard them.	
——	——	——	48. Cover the patient and help the patient to a position of comfort.	
——	——	——	49. Place the bed in the lowest position; elevate rails as needed.	
——	——	——	50. Return the thermometer to the charging unit.	

Skill Checklists for Fundamentals of Nursing:
The Art and Science of Person-Centered Nursing Care, 8th edition

Name _____   Date _____

Unit _____   Position _____

Instructor/Evaluator: _____   Position _____

SKILL 24-2
Assessing a Peripheral Pulse by Palpation

Goal: The patient's pulse is assessed accurately without injury and the patient experiences only minimal discomfort.

Columns: Excellent | Satisfactory | Needs Practice | | Comments

1. Check medical order or nursing care plan for frequency of pulse assessment. More frequent pulse measurement may be appropriate based on nursing judgment.
2. Perform hand hygiene and put on PPE, if indicated.
3. Identify the patient.
4. Close the curtains around the bed and close the door to the room, if possible. Discuss the procedure with the patient and assess the patient's ability to assist with the procedure.
5. Put on gloves, if indicated.
6. Select the appropriate peripheral site based on assessment data.
7. Move the patient's clothing to expose only the site chosen.
8. Place your first, second, and third fingers over the artery. *Lightly compress the artery so pulsations can be felt and counted.*
9. Using a watch with a second hand; count the number of pulsations felt for 30 seconds. Multiply this number by 2 to calculate the rate for 1 minute. *If the rate, rhythm, or amplitude of the pulse is abnormal in any way, palpate and count the pulse for 1 minute.*
10. Note the rhythm and amplitude of the pulse.
11. When measurement is completed, remove gloves, if worn. Cover the patient and help the patient to a position of comfort.
12. Remove additional PPE, if used. Perform hand hygiene.

Skill Checklists for Fundamentals of Nursing:
The Art and Science of Person-Centered Nursing Care, 8th edition

Name _____ Date _____

Unit _____ Position _____

Instructor/Evaluator: _____ Position _____

SKILL 24-3
Assessing Respiration

Goal: The patient's respirations are assessed accurately without injury and the patient experiences only minimal discomfort.

Columns: Excellent | Satisfactory | Needs Practice | | Comments

1. *While your fingers are still in place for the pulse measurement, after counting the pulse rate, observe the patient's respirations.*

2. Note the rise and fall of the patient's chest.

3. Using a watch with a second hand, count the number of respirations for 30 seconds. Multiply this number by 2 to calculate the respiratory rate per minute.

4. *If respirations are abnormal in any way, count the respirations for at least 1 full minute.*

5. Note the depth and rhythm of the respirations.

6. When measurement is completed, remove gloves, if worn. Cover the patient and help the patient to a position of comfort.

7. Remove additional PPE, if used. Perform hand hygiene.

Skill Checklists for Fundamentals of Nursing:
The Art and Science of Person-Centered Nursing Care, 8th edition

Name _____   Date _____

Unit _____   Position _____

Instructor/Evaluator: _____   Position _____

SKILL 24-4

Assessing Blood Pressure by Auscultation

Goal: The patient's blood pressure is measured accurately with minimal discomfort to the patient.

Excellent	Satisfactory	Needs Practice		Comments
___	___	___	1. Check the medical order or nursing care plan for frequency of blood pressure measurement. More frequent measurement may be appropriate based on nursing judgment.	
___	___	___	2. Perform hand hygiene and put on PPE, if indicated.	
___	___	___	3. Identify the patient.	
___	___	___	4. Close the curtains around the bed and close the door to the room, if possible. Discuss procedure with the patient and assess the patient's ability to assist with the procedure. Validate that the patient has relaxed for several minutes.	
___	___	___	5. Put on gloves, if indicated.	
___	___	___	6. Select the appropriate arm for application of the cuff.	
___	___	___	7. Have the patient assume a comfortable lying or sitting position with the forearm supported at the level of the heart and the palm of the hand upward. If the measurement is taken in the supine position, support the arm with a pillow. In the sitting position, support the arm yourself or by using the bedside table. If the patient is sitting, have the patient sit back in the chair so that the chair supports the patient's back. In addition, make sure the patient keeps the legs uncrossed.	
___	___	___	8. Expose the brachial artery by removing garments or move a sleeve, if it is not too tight, above the area where the cuff will be placed.	
___	___	___	9. Palpate the location of the brachial artery. *Center the bladder of the cuff over the brachial artery, about midway on the arm, so that the lower edge of the cuff is about 2.5 to 5 cm (1 to 2 inches) above the inner aspect of the elbow. Line up the artery marking on the cuff with the patient's brachial artery.* The tubing should extend from the edge of the cuff nearer the patient's elbow.	
___	___	___	10. Wrap the cuff around the arm smoothly and snugly, and fasten it. Do not allow any clothing to interfere with the proper placement of the cuff.	
___	___	___	11. Check that the needle on the aneroid gauge is within the zero mark. If using a mercury manometer, check to see that the manometer is in the vertical position and that the mercury is within the zero level with the gauge at eye level.	

Excellent	Satisfactory	Needs Practice	

Assessing Blood Pressure by Auscultation *(Continued)*

				Comments

Estimating Systolic Pressure

—— —— —— 12. Palpate the pulse at the brachial or radial artery by pressing gently with the fingertips.

—— —— —— 13. Tighten the screw valve on the air pump.

—— —— —— 14. *Inflate the cuff while continuing to palpate the artery. Note the point on the gauge where the pulse disappears.*

—— —— —— 15. Deflate the cuff and wait 1 minute.

Obtaining Blood Pressure Measurement

—— —— —— 16. Assume a position that is no more than 3 feet away from the gauge.

—— —— —— 17. Place the stethoscope earpieces in your ears. Direct the earpieces forward into the canal and not against the ear itself.

—— —— —— 18. Place the bell or diaphragm of the stethoscope firmly but with as little pressure as possible over the brachial artery. Do not allow the stethoscope to touch clothing or the cuff.

—— —— —— 19. Pump the pressure 30 mm Hg above the point at which the systolic pressure was palpated and estimated. Open the valve on the manometer and allow air to escape slowly (allowing the gauge to drop 2 to 3 mm per second).

—— —— —— 20. *Note the point on the gauge at which the first faint, but clear, sound appears that slowly increases in intensity. Note this number as the systolic pressure. Read the pressure to the closest 2 mm Hg.*

—— —— —— 21. Do not reinflate the cuff once the air is being released to recheck the systolic pressure reading.

—— —— —— 22. *Note the point at which the sound completely disappears. Note this number as the diastolic pressure. Read the pressure to the closest 2 mm Hg.*

—— —— —— 23. Allow the remaining air to escape quickly. Repeat any suspicious reading, but wait at least 1 minute. Deflate the cuff completely between attempts to check the blood pressure.

—— —— —— 24. When measurement is completed, remove the cuff. Remove gloves, if worn. Cover the patient and help the patient to a position of comfort.

—— —— —— 25. Clean the bell or diaphragm of the stethoscope with the alcohol wipe. Clean and store the sphygmomanometer, according to facility policy.

—— —— —— 26. Remove additional PPE, if used. Perform hand hygiene.

Skill Checklists for Fundamentals of Nursing:
The Art and Science of Person-Centered Nursing Care, 8th edition

Name _____   Date _____

Unit _____   Position _____

Instructor/Evaluator: _____   Position _____

SKILL 25-1
Using a Bed Scale

Goal: The patient's weight is assessed accurately, without injury, and the patient experiences minimal discomfort.

Excellent	Satisfactory	Needs Practice		Comments
——	——	——	1. Check the medical order or nursing plan of care for frequency of weight measurement. More frequent measurement of the patient's weight may be appropriate based on nursing judgment. Obtain the assistance of a second caregiver, based on the patient's mobility and ability to cooperate with the procedure.	
——	——	——	2. Perform hand hygiene and put on PPE, if indicated.	
——	——	——	3. Identify the patient.	
——	——	——	4. Close curtains around the bed and close the door to the room if possible. Discuss the procedure with the patient and assess the patient's ability to assist with the procedure.	
——	——	——	5. Place a cover over the sling of the bed scale.	
——	——	——	6. Attach the sling to the bed scale. Lay the sheet or bath blanket in the sling. Turn the scale on. ***Balance the scale so that weight reads 0.0.***	
——	——	——	7. Adjust the bed to a comfortable working position, usually elbow height of the caregiver (VISN 8, 2012). Position one caregiver on each side of the bed if two caregivers are present. Raise side rail on the opposite side of the bed from where the scale is located, if not already in place. Cover the patient with the sheet or bath blanket. Remove other covers and any pillows.	
——	——	——	8. Turn the patient onto his or her side facing the side rail, keeping the patient's body covered with the sheet or blanket. Remove the sling from the scale. Place the cover on the sling. Roll the cover and sling lengthwise. Place the rolled sling under the patient, making sure the patient is centered in the sling.	
——	——	——	9. Roll the patient back over the sling and onto the other side. Pull the sling through, as if placing the sheet under the patient, unrolling the sling as it is pulled through.	
——	——	——	10. Roll the scale over the bed so that the arms of the scale are directly over the patient. ***Spread the base of the scale.*** Lower the arms of the scale and place the arm hooks into the holes on the sling.	

SKILL 25-1

Using a Bed Scale *(Continued)*

Excellent	Satisfactory	Needs Practice		Comments
——	——	——	11. Once the scale arms are hooked onto the sling, gradually elevate the sling so that the patient is lifted up off of the bed. *Assess all tubes and drains, making sure that none have tension placed on them as the scale is lifted. Once the sling is no longer touching the bed, ensure that nothing else is hanging onto the sling (e.g., ventilator or IV tubing). If any tubing is connected to the patient, raise it up so that it is not adding any weight to the patient.*	
——	——	——	12. Note the weight reading on the scale. Slowly and gently, lower the patient back onto the bed. Disconnect the scale arms from the sling. Close the base of the scale and pull it away from the bed.	
——	——	——	13. Raise the side rail. Turn the patient to the side rail. Roll the sling up against the patient's backside.	
——	——	——	14. Raise the other side rail. Roll the patient back over the sling and up, facing the other side rail. Remove the sling from the bed. Remove gloves, if used. Raise the remaining side rail.	
——	——	——	15. Cover the patient and help him or her to a position of comfort. Place the bed in the lowest position.	
——	——	——	16. Remove the disposable cover from the sling and discard in the appropriate receptacle.	
——	——	——	17. Remove additional PPE, if used. Clean equipment based on facility policy. Perform hand hygiene.	
——	——	——	18. Replace the scale and sling in the appropriate spot. Plug the scale into the electrical outlet.	

Skill Checklists for Fundamentals of Nursing:
The Art and Science of Person-Centered Nursing Care, 8th edition

Name _____ Date _____

Unit _____ Position _____

Instructor/Evaluator: _____ Position _____

SKILL 25-2

Assessing the Neurologic, Musculoskeletal, and Peripheral Vascular Systems

Goal: The assessments are completed without causing the patient to experience anxiety or discomfort, the findings are documented, and the appropriate referral is made to other health care professionals, as needed, for further evaluation.

Excellent	Satisfactory	Needs Practice		Comments
___	___	___	1. Perform hand hygiene and put on PPE, if indicated.	
___	___	___	2. Identify the patient.	
___	___	___	3. Close the curtains around the bed and close the door to the room, if possible. Explain the purpose of the neurologic, musculoskeletal, and peripheral vascular examinations and what you are going to do. Answer any questions.	
			4. Help the patient undress, if needed, and provide a patient gown. Assist the patient to a supine position, if possible. Use the bath blanket to cover any exposed area other than the one being assessed.	
___	___	___	5. Begin with a survey of the patient's overall hygiene and physical appearance.	
___	___	___	6. Assess the patient's mental status.	
___	___	___	a. Evaluate the patient's orientation to person, place, and time.	
___	___	___	b. Evaluate level of consciousness.	
___	___	___	c. Assess memory (immediate recall and past memory).	
___	___	___	d. Assess abstract reasoning by asking the patient to explain a proverb, such as "The early bird catches the worm."	
___	___	___	e. Evaluate the patient's ability to understand the spoken and written word.	
___	___	___	7. Test cranial nerve (CN) function.	
___	___	___	a. Ask the patient to close the eyes, occlude one nostril, and then identify the smell of different substances, such as coffee, chocolate, or alcohol. Repeat with the other nostril.	
___	___	___	b. Test visual acuity and pupillary constriction. Refer to the previous discussion in the assessment of the head and neck.	
___	___	___	c. Move the patient's eyes through the six cardinal positions of gaze. Refer to previous discussion in the assessment of the head and neck.	

SKILL 25-2

Assessing the Neurologic, Musculoskeletal, and Peripheral Vascular Systems *(Continued)*

Excellent	Satisfactory	Needs Practice		Comments

			d. Ask the patient to smile, frown, wrinkle the forehead, and puff out cheeks.	
			e. Ask the patient to protrude the tongue and push against the cheek with the tongue.	
			f. Palpate the jaw muscles. Ask the patient to open and clench jaws. Stroke the patients face with a cotton ball.	
			g. Test hearing with the whispered voice test. Refer to previous discussion in the assessment of the head and neck.	
			h. Put on gloves. Ask the patient to open the mouth. While observing the soft palate, ask the patient to say "ah"; observe upward movement of the soft palate. Test the gag reflex by touching the posterior pharynx with the tongue depressor. Explain to patient that this may be uncomfortable. Ask the patient to swallow. Remove gloves.	
			i. Place your hands on the patient's shoulders while he or she shrugs against resistance. Then place your hand on the patient's left cheek, then the right cheek, and have the patient push against it.	
			8. Check the patient's ability to move his or her neck. Ask the patient to touch the chin to the chest and to each shoulder, then move each ear to the corresponding shoulder, and then tip the head back as far as possible.	
			9. Inspect the upper extremities. Observe for skin color, presence of lesions, rashes, and muscle mass. Palpate for skin temperature, texture, and presence of masses.	
			10. Ask the patient to extend the arms forward and then rapidly turn the palms up and down.	
			11. Ask the patient to flex the upper arm and to resist the examiner's opposing force.	
			12. Inspect and palpate the hands, fingers, wrists, and elbow joints.	
			13. Ask the patient to bend and straighten the elbow, and flex and extend the wrists and hands.	
			14. Palpate the skin and the radial and brachial pulses. Assess the pulse rate, quality or amplitude, and rhythm. Test capillary refill.	
			15. Have the patient squeeze two of your fingers.	

Excellent	Satisfactory	Needs Practice	SKILL 25-2 **Assessing the Neurologic, Musculoskeletal, and Peripheral Vascular Systems** *(Continued)*	Comments
——	——	——	16. Ask the patient to close the eyes. Using your finger or applicator, trace a one-digit number on the patient's palm and ask the patient to identify the number. Repeat on the other hand with a different number.	
——	——	——	17. Ask the patient to close the eyes. Place a familiar object, such as a key, in the patient's hand and ask the patient to identify the object. Repeat using another object for the other hand.	
——	——	——	18. Assist the patient to a supine position. Palpate and then use the bell of the stethoscope to auscultate the femoral pulses in the groin, if not done during assessment of the abdomen. Note the strength of the pulse and grade it as with peripheral pulses.	
——	——	——	19. Examine the lower extremities. Inspect the legs and feet for color, lesions, varicosities, hair growth, nail growth, edema, and muscle mass.	
——	——	——	20. Assess for pitting edema in the lower extremities by pressing fingers into the skin at the pretibial area and dorsum of the foot. If an indentation remains in the skin after the fingers have been lifted, pitting edema is present.	
——	——	——	21. Palpate for pulses and skin temperature at the posterior tibial, dorsalis pedis, and popliteal areas. Assess the pulse rate, quality or amplitude, and rhythm. Test capillary refill.	
——	——	——	22. Have the patient perform the straight leg test with one leg at a time.	
——	——	——	23. Ask the patient to move one leg laterally with the knee straight to test abduction and medially to test adduction of the hips.	
——	——	——	24. Ask the patient to raise the thigh against the resistance of your hand; next have the patient push outward against the resistance of your hand; then have the patient pull backward against the resistance of your hand. Repeat on the opposite side.	
——	——	——	25. Test plantar reflex. Stroke the sole of the patient's foot with the end of a hard object such as the edge of a tongue depressor or a key. Begin at the heel and apply firm but gentle pressure to the lateral aspect of the foot. Continue to the base of the toes. Repeat on the other side.	
——	——	——	26. Ask patient to dorsiflex and then plantarflex both feet against opposing resistance.	

SKILL 25-2

Assessing the Neurologic, Musculoskeletal, and Peripheral Vascular Systems (Continued)

Excellent	Satisfactory	Needs Practice		Comments
——	——	——	27. As needed, assist the patient to a standing position. Observe the patient as he or she walks with a regular gait, on the toes, on the heels, and then heel to toe.	
——	——	——	28. Perform the Romberg test; ask the patient to stand straight with feet together, both eyes closed with arms at side. Wait 20 seconds and observe for patient swaying and ability to maintain balance. Be alert to prevent patient fall or injury related to losing balance during this assessment.	
——	——	——	29. Assist the patient to a comfortable position.	
——	——	——	30. Remove PPE, if used. Perform hand hygiene. Continue with assessments of specific body systems, as appropriate, or indicated. Initiate appropriate referral to other health care practitioners for further evaluation, as indicated.	

5 by Wolters Kluwer. *Skill Checklists for Fundamentals of Nursing: The Art and* n-*Centered Nursing Care*, 8th edition, by Carol Taylor, Carol Lillis, and Pamela Lynn.

Skill Checklists for Fundamentals of Nursing:
The Art and Science of Person-Centered Nursing Care, 8th edition

Name _____ Date _____

Unit _____ Position _____

Instructor/Evaluator: _____ Position _____

Excellent	Satisfactory	Needs Practice		Comments

SKILL 28-1

Administering Oral Medications

Goal: The patient will swallow the prescribed medication at the proper time.

1. Gather equipment. Check each medication order against the original in the medical record, according to facility policy. Clarify any inconsistencies. Check the patient's medical record for allergies.

2. Know the actions, special nursing considerations, safe dose ranges, purpose of administration, and adverse effects of the medications to be administered. Consider the appropriateness of the medication for this patient.

3. Perform hand hygiene.

4. Move the medication cart to the outside of the patient's room or prepare for administration in the medication area.

5. Unlock the medication cart or drawer. Enter the pass code into the computer and scan employee identification, if required.

6. *Prepare medications for one patient at a time.*

7. Read the CMAR/MAR and select the proper medication from the unit stock or patient's medication drawer.

8. Compare the medication label with the CMAR/MAR. Check expiration dates and perform calculations, if necessary. Scan the bar code on the package, if required.

9. Prepare the required medications:

   a. *Unit dose packages:* Place unit dose-packaged medications in a disposable cup. ***Do not open the wrapper until at the bedside.*** Keep opioids and medications that require special nursing assessments in a separate container.

   b. *Multidose containers:* When removing tablets or capsules from a multidose bottle, pour the necessary number into the bottle cap and then place the tablets or capsules in a medication cup. Break only scored tablets, if necessary, to obtain the proper dosage. Do not touch tablets or capsules with hands.

SKILL 28-1

Administering Oral Medications *(Continued)*

Excellent	Satisfactory	Needs Practice		Comments
——	——	——	c. *Liquid medication in multidose bottle:* When pouring liquid medications out of a multidose bottle, hold the bottle so that the label is against the palm. Use the appropriate measuring device when pouring liquids, and read the amount of medication at the bottom of the meniscus at eye level. Wipe the lip of the bottle with a paper towel.	
——	——	——	10. *Depending on facility policy, the third check of the label may occur at this point. If so, when all medications for one patient have been prepared, recheck the labels with the CMAR/MAR before taking the medications to the patient.*	
——	——	——	11. Replace any multidose containers in the patient's drawer or unit stock. *Lock the medication cart before leaving it.*	
——	——	——	12. Transport medications to the patient's bedside carefully, and keep the medications in sight at all times.	
——	——	——	13. *Ensure that the patient receives the medications at the correct time.*	
——	——	——	14. Perform hand hygiene and put on PPE, if indicated.	
——	——	——	15. *Identify the patient. Compare the information with the CMAR/MAR. The patient should be identified using at least two methods:*	
——	——	——	a. Check the name on the patient's identification band.	
——	——	——	b. Check the identification number on the patient's identification band.	
——	——	——	c. Check the birth date on the patient's identification band.	
——	——	——	d. Ask the patient to state name and birth date, based on facility policy.	
——	——	——	16. *Complete necessary assessments before administering medications. Check the patient's allergy bracelet or ask the patient about allergies. Explain the purpose and action of each medication to the patient.*	
——	——	——	17. Scan the patient's bar code on the identification band, if required.	
——	——	——	18. *Based on facility policy, the third check of the medication label may occur at this point. If so, recheck the labels with the CMAR/MAR before administering the medications to the patient.*	
——	——	——	19. Assist the patient to an upright or lateral (side-lying) position.	

Excellent	Satisfactory	Needs Practice		Comments
			SKILL 28-1 **Administering Oral Medications** *(Continued)*	
——	——	——	20. Administer medications:	
——	——	——	a. Offer water or other permitted fluids with pills, capsules, tablets, and some liquid medications.	
——	——	——	b. Ask whether the patient prefers to take the medications by hand or in a cup.	
——	——	——	21. *Remain with the patient until each medication is swallowed. Never leave medication at the patient's bedside.*	
——	——	——	22. Assist the patient to a comfortable position. Remove PPE, if used. Perform hand hygiene.	
——	——	——	23. Document the administration of the medication immediately after administration.	
——	——	——	24. Evaluate the patient's response to medication within the appropriate time frame.	

Skill Checklists for Fundamentals of Nursing:
The Art and Science of Person-Centered Nursing Care, 8th edition

Name _____ Date _____

Unit _____ Position _____

Instructor/Evaluator: _____ Position _____

SKILL 28-2
Removing Medication From an Ampule

Goal: The proper dose of medication will be removed in a sterile manner, and will be free from glass shards.

Excellent	Satisfactory	Needs Practice		Comments
⎯⎯	⎯⎯	⎯⎯	1. Gather equipment. Check the medication order against the original order in the medical record, according to facility policy. Clarify any inconsistencies. Check the patient's chart for allergies.	
⎯⎯	⎯⎯	⎯⎯	2. Know the actions, special nursing considerations, safe dose ranges, purpose of administration, and adverse effects of the medications to be administered. Consider the appropriateness of the medication for this patient.	
⎯⎯	⎯⎯	⎯⎯	3. Perform hand hygiene.	
⎯⎯	⎯⎯	⎯⎯	4. Move the medication cart to the outside of the patient's room or prepare for administration in the medication area.	
⎯⎯	⎯⎯	⎯⎯	5. Unlock the medication cart or drawer. Enter the pass code and scan employee identification, if required.	
⎯⎯	⎯⎯	⎯⎯	6. *Prepare medications for one patient at a time.*	
⎯⎯	⎯⎯	⎯⎯	7. Read the CMAR/MAR and select the proper medication from unit stock or the patient's medication drawer.	
⎯⎯	⎯⎯	⎯⎯	8. Compare the label with the CMAR/MAR. Check expiration dates and perform calculations, if necessary. Scan the bar code on the package, if required.	
⎯⎯	⎯⎯	⎯⎯	9. Tap the stem of the ampule or twist your wrist quickly while holding the ampule vertically.	
⎯⎯	⎯⎯	⎯⎯	10. Wrap a small gauze pad around the neck of the ampule.	
⎯⎯	⎯⎯	⎯⎯	11. Use a snapping motion to break off the top of the ampule along the scored line at its neck. *Always break away from your body.*	
⎯⎯	⎯⎯	⎯⎯	12. Attach the filter needle to the syringe. Remove the cap from the filter needle by pulling it straight off.	
⎯⎯	⎯⎯	⎯⎯	13. Withdraw medication in the amount ordered plus a small amount more (approximately 30% more). *Do not inject air into the solution. While inserting the filter needle into the ampule, be careful not to touch the rim.* Use either of the following methods to withdraw the medication:	
⎯⎯	⎯⎯	⎯⎯	a. Insert the tip of the needle into the ampule, which is upright on a flat surface, and withdraw fluid into the syringe. *Touch the plunger at the knob only.*	

SKILL 28-2

Removing Medication From an Ampule *(Continued)*

Excellent	Satisfactory	Needs Practice		Comments
——	——	——	b. Insert the tip of the needle into the ampule and invert the ampule. Keep the needle centered and not touching the sides of the ampule. Withdraw fluid into syringe. *Touch the plunger at the knob only.*	
——	——	——	14. Wait until the needle has been withdrawn to tap the syringe and expel the air carefully by pushing on the plunger. *Check the amount of medication in the syringe with the medication dose and discard any surplus according to facility policy.*	
——	——	——	15. *Depending on facility policy, the third check of the label may occur at this point. If so, when all medications for one patient have been prepared, recheck the labels with the CMAR/MAR before taking the medications to the patient.*	
——	——	——	16. *Engage the safety guard on the filter needle and remove the needle. Discard the filter needle in a suitable container. Attach the appropriate administration device to the syringe.*	
——	——	——	17. Discard the ampule in a suitable container.	
——	——	——	18. Lock the medication cart before leaving it.	
——	——	——	19. Perform hand hygiene.	
——	——	——	20. Proceed with administration, based on the prescribed route.	

Skill Checklists for Fundamentals of Nursing:
The Art and Science of Person-Centered Nursing Care, 8th edition

Name _____ Date _____

Unit _____ Position _____

Instructor/Evaluator: _____ Position _____

SKILL 28-3
Removing Medication From a Vial

Goal: The proper dosage of medication is withdrawn into a syringe using sterile technique.

Excellent	Satisfactory	Needs Practice		Comments
___	___	___	1. Gather equipment. Check the medication order against the original order in the medical record, according to facility policy. Clarify any inconsistencies. Check the patient's chart for allergies.	
___	___	___	2. Know the actions, special nursing considerations, safe dose ranges, purpose of administration, and adverse effects of the medications to be administered. Consider the appropriateness of the medication for this patient.	
___	___	___	3. Perform hand hygiene.	
___	___	___	4. Move the medication cart to the outside of the patient's room or prepare for administration in the medication area.	
___	___	___	5. Unlock the medication cart or drawer. Enter pass code and scan employee identification, if required.	
___	___	___	6. *Prepare medications for one patient at a time.*	
___	___	___	7. Read the CMAR/MAR and select the proper medication from unit stock or the patient's medication drawer.	
___	___	___	8. Compare the label with the CMAR/MAR. Check expiration dates and perform calculations, if necessary. Scan the bar code on the package, if required.	
___	___	___	9. Remove the metal or plastic cap on the vial that protects the rubber stopper.	
___	___	___	10. *Swab the rubber top with the antimicrobial swab and allow to dry.*	
___	___	___	11. Remove the cap from the needle or blunt cannula by pulling it straight off. Touch the plunger at the knob only. Draw back an amount of air into the syringe that is equal to the specific dose of medication to be withdrawn. Some facilities require use of a filter needle when withdrawing premixed medication from multidose vials.	
___	___	___	12. Hold the vial on a flat surface. Pierce the rubber stopper in the center with the needle tip and inject the measured air into the space above the solution. Do not inject air into the solution.	
___	___	___	13. Invert the vial. *Keep the tip of the needle or blunt cannula below the fluid level.*	

Removing Medication From a Vial (Continued)

Excellent	Satisfactory	Needs Practice		Comments
___	___	___	14. Hold the vial in one hand and use the other to withdraw the medication. *Touch the plunger at the knob only. Draw up the prescribed amount of medication while holding the syringe vertically and at eye level.*	
___	___	___	15. If any air bubbles accumulate in the syringe, tap the barrel of the syringe sharply and move the needle past the fluid into the air space to reinject the air bubble into the vial. Return the needle tip to the solution and continue withdrawal of the medication.	
___	___	___	16. After the correct dose is withdrawn, remove the needle from the vial and carefully replace the cap over the needle. *If a filter needle has been used to draw up the medication, remove it and attach the appropriate administration device.* Some facilities require changing the needle, if one was used to withdraw the medication, before administering the medication.	
___	___	___	17. *Check the amount of medication in the syringe with the medication dose and discard any surplus.*	
___	___	___	18. *Depending on facility policy, the third check of the label may occur at this point. If so, when all medications for one patient have been prepared, recheck the labels with the CMAR/MAR before taking the medications to the patient.*	
___	___	___	19. *If a multidose vial is being used, label the vial with the date and time opened, and store the vial containing the remaining medication according to facility policy.*	
___	___	___	20. Lock the medication cart before leaving it.	
___	___	___	21. Perform hand hygiene.	
___	___	___	22. Proceed with administration, based on the prescribed route.	

Skill Checklists for Fundamentals of Nursing:
The Art and Science of Person-Centered Nursing Care, 8th edition

Name _____   Date _____

Unit _____   Position _____

Instructor/Evaluator: _____   Position _____

Excellent	Satisfactory	Needs Practice	SKILL 28-4 **Mixing Medications From Two Vials in One Syringe**	Comments
			Goal: The proper dosage of medication is withdrawn into a syringe using sterile technique.	
____	____	____	1. Gather equipment. Check the medication order against the original order in the medical record, according to facility policy.	
____	____	____	2. Know the actions, special nursing considerations, safe dose ranges, purpose of administration, and adverse effects of the medications to be administered. Consider the appropriateness of the medication for this patient.	
____	____	____	3. Perform hand hygiene.	
____	____	____	4. Move the medication cart to the outside of the patient's room or prepare for administration in the medication area.	
____	____	____	5. Unlock the medication cart or drawer. Enter the pass code and scan employee identification, if required.	
____	____	____	6. *Prepare medications for one patient at a time.*	
____	____	____	7. Read the CMAR/MAR and select the proper medications from unit stock or the patient's medication drawer.	
____	____	____	8. Compare the labels with the CMAR/MAR. Check expiration dates and perform dosage calculations, if necessary. Scan the bar code on the package, if required.	
____	____	____	9. If necessary, remove the cap that protects the rubber stopper on each vial.	
____	____	____	10. *If medication is a suspension (e.g., a modified insulin, such as NPH insulin), roll and agitate the vial to mix it well.*	
____	____	____	11. *Cleanse the rubber tops with antimicrobial swabs.* Allow the top to dry.	
____	____	____	12. Remove the cap from the needle by pulling it straight off. Touch the plunger at the knob only. Draw back an amount of air into the syringe that is equal to the dose of modified insulin to be withdrawn.	
____	____	____	13. Hold the modified vial on a flat surface. Pierce the rubber stopper in the center with the needle tip and inject the measured air into the space above the solution. Do not inject air into the solution. Withdraw the needle.	
____	____	____	14. Draw back an amount of air into the syringe that is equal to the dose of unmodified insulin to be withdrawn.	

SKILL 28-4

Mixing Medications From Two Vials in One Syringe (Continued)

Excellent	Satisfactory	Needs Practice		Comments
——	——	——	15. Hold the unmodified vial on a flat surface. Pierce the rubber stopper in the center with the needle tip and inject the measured air into the space above the solution. Do not inject air into the solution. Keep the needle in the vial.	
——	——	——	16. Invert the vial of unmodified insulin. Hold the vial in one hand and use the other to withdraw the medication. *Touch the plunger at the knob only. Draw up the prescribed amount of medication while holding the syringe at eye level and vertically.* Turn the vial over, then remove the needle from the vial.	
——	——	——	17. Check that there are no air bubbles in the syringe.	
——	——	——	18. *Check the amount of medication in the syringe with the medication dose and discard any surplus.*	
——	——	——	19. *Recheck the vial label with the CMAR/MAR.*	
——	——	——	20. Calculate the endpoint on the syringe for the combined insulin amount by adding the number of units for each dose together.	
——	——	——	21. Insert the needle into the modified vial and invert it, taking care not to push the plunger and inject medication from the syringe into the vial. Invert the vial of modified insulin. Hold the vial in one hand and use the other to withdraw the medication. *Touch the plunger at the knob only. Draw up the prescribed amount of medication while holding the syringe at eye level and vertically. Take care to withdraw only the prescribed amount.* Turn the vial over, then remove the needle from the vial. Carefully recap the needle. Carefully replace the cap over the needle.	
——	——	——	22. *Check the amount of medication in the syringe with the medication dose.*	
——	——	——	23. *Depending on facility policy, the third check of the label may occur at this point. If so, recheck the label with the CMAR/MAR before taking the medications to the patient.*	
——	——	——	24. *Label the vials with the date and time opened, and store the vials containing the remaining medication according to facility policy.*	
——	——	——	25. Lock the medication cart before leaving it.	
——	——	——	26. Perform hand hygiene.	
——	——	——	27. Proceed with administration, based on the prescribed route.	

34

Name _____   Date _____

Unit _____   Position _____

Instructor/Evaluator: _____   Position _____

SKILL 28-5

Administering an Intradermal Injection

Goal: Medication is safely injected intradermally causing a wheal to appear at the site of the injection.

Excellent	Satisfactory	Needs Practice		Comments
___	___	___	1. Gather equipment. Check each medication order against the original order in the medical record according to facility policy. Clarify any inconsistencies. Check the patient's chart for allergies.	
___	___	___	2. Know the actions, special nursing considerations, safe dose ranges, purpose of administration, and adverse effects of the medications to be administered. Consider the appropriateness of the medication for this patient.	
___	___	___	3. Perform hand hygiene.	
___	___	___	4. Move the medication cart to the outside of the patient's room or prepare for administration in the medication area.	
___	___	___	5. Unlock the medication cart or drawer. Enter the pass code and scan employee identification, if required.	
___	___	___	6. *Prepare medications for one patient at a time.*	
___	___	___	7. Read the CMAR/MAR and select the proper medication from unit stock or the patient's medication drawer.	
___	___	___	8. Compare the label with the CMAR/MAR. Check expiration dates and perform calculations, if necessary. Scan the bar code on the package, if required.	
___	___	___	9. If necessary, withdraw medication from an ampule or vial.	
___	___	___	10. *Depending on facility policy, the third check of the label may occur at this point. If so, when all medications for one patient have been prepared, recheck the labels with the CMAR/MAR before taking the medications to the patient.*	
___	___	___	11. Lock the medication cart before leaving it.	
___	___	___	12. Transport medications to the patient's bedside carefully, and keep the medications in sight at all times.	
___	___	___	13. *Ensure that the patient receives the medications at the correct time.*	
___	___	___	14. Perform hand hygiene and put on PPE, if indicated.	

Excellent	**Satisfactory**	**Needs Practice**	

SKILL 28-5
Administering an Intradermal Injection *(Continued)*

Comments

Excellent	Satisfactory	Needs Practice	
——	——	——	15. *Identify the patient. Compare the information with the CMAR/MAR. The patient should be identified using at least two methods:*
——	——	——	a. Check the name on the patient's identification band.
——	——	——	b. Check the identification number on the patient's identification band.
——	——	——	c. Check the birth date on the patient's identification band.
——	——	——	d. Ask the patient to state his or her name and birth date, based on facility policy.
——	——	——	16. Close the door to the room or pull the bedside curtain.
——	——	——	17. *Complete necessary assessments before administering medications. Check the allergy bracelet or ask the patient about allergies. Explain the purpose and action of the medication to the patient.*
——	——	——	18. Scan the patient's bar code on the identification band, if required.
——	——	——	19. *Based on facility policy, the third check of the label may occur at this point. If so, recheck the labels with the CMAR/MAR before administering the medications to the patient.*
——	——	——	20. Put on clean gloves.
——	——	——	21. Select an appropriate administration site. Assist the patient to the appropriate position for the site chosen. Drape as needed to expose only the area of the site to be used.
——	——	——	22. Cleanse the site with an antimicrobial swab while wiping with a firm, circular motion and moving outward from the injection site. Allow the skin to dry.
——	——	——	23. Remove the needle cap with the nondominant hand by pulling it straight off.
——	——	——	24. Use the nondominant hand to spread the skin taut over the injection site.
——	——	——	25. Hold the syringe in the dominant hand, between the thumb and forefinger with the bevel of the needle up.
——	——	——	26. Hold the syringe at a 5- to 15-degree angle from the site. Place the needle almost flat against the patient's skin, bevel side up, and insert the needle into the skin. Insert the needle only about ⅛ inch with entire bevel under the skin.
——	——	——	27. Once the needle is in place, steady the lower end of the syringe. Slide your dominant hand to the end of the plunger.

SKILL 28-5

Administering an Intradermal Injection *(Continued)*

Excellent	Satisfactory	Needs Practice		Comments
——	——	——	28. Slowly inject the agent while watching for a small wheal or blister to appear.	
——	——	——	29. Withdraw the needle quickly at the same angle that it was inserted. Do not recap the used needle. Engage the safety shield or needle guard.	
——	——	——	30. *Do not massage the area after removing the needle. Tell the patient not to rub or scratch the site. If necessary, gently blot the site with a dry gauze square. Do not apply pressure or rub the site.*	
——	——	——	31. Assist the patient to a position of comfort.	
——	——	——	32. Discard the needle and syringe in the appropriate receptacle.	
——	——	——	33. Remove gloves and additional PPE, if used. Perform hand hygiene.	
——	——	——	34. Document the administration of the medication immediately after administration.	
——	——	——	35. Evaluate the patient's response to the medication within the appropriate time frame.	
——	——	——	36. Observe the area for signs of a reaction at determined intervals after administration. Inform the patient of the need for inspection.	

Skill Checklists for Fundamentals of Nursing:
The Art and Science of Person-Centered Nursing Care, 8th edition

Name _____   Date _____

Unit _____   Position _____

Instructor/Evaluator: _____   Position _____

SKILL 28-6

Administering a Subcutaneous Injection

Goal: The patient safely receives medication via the subcutaneous route.

Excellent	Satisfactory	Needs Practice		Comments
___	___	___	1. Gather equipment. Check each medication order against the original order in the medical record, according to facility policy. Clarify any inconsistencies. Check the patient's chart for allergies.	
___	___	___	2. Know the actions, special nursing considerations, safe dose ranges, purpose of administration, and adverse effects of the medications to be administered. Consider the appropriateness of the medication for this patient.	
___	___	___	3. Perform hand hygiene.	
___	___	___	4. Move the medication cart to the outside of the patient's room or prepare for administration in the medication area.	
___	___	___	5. Unlock the medication cart or drawer. Enter the pass code and scan employee identification, if required.	
___	___	___	6. *Prepare medications for one patient at a time.*	
___	___	___	7. Read the CMAR/MAR and select the proper medication from unit stock or the patient's medication drawer.	
___	___	___	8. Compare the label with the CMAR/MAR. Check expiration dates and perform calculations, if necessary. Scan the bar code on the package, if required.	
___	___	___	9. If necessary, withdraw medication from an ampule or vial.	
___	___	___	10. *Depending on facility policy, the third check of the label may occur at this point. If so, when all medications for one patient have been prepared, recheck the labels with the CMAR/MAR before taking the medications to the patient.*	
___	___	___	11. Lock the medication cart before leaving it.	
___	___	___	12. Transport medications to the patient's bedside carefully, and keep the medications in sight at all times.	
___	___	___	13. *Ensure that the patient receives the medications at the correct time.*	
___	___	___	14. Perform hand hygiene and put on PPE, if indicated.	

SKILL 28-6

Administering a Subcutaneous Injection *(Continued)*

Excellent	Satisfactory	Needs Practice		Comments
___	___	___	15. *Identify the patient. Compare the information with the CMAR/MAR. The patient should be identified using at least two methods:*	
___	___	___	a. Check the name on the patient's identification band.	
___	___	___	b. Check the identification number on the patient's identification band.	
___	___	___	c. Check the birth date on the patient's identification band.	
___	___	___	d. Ask the patient to state his or her name and birth date, based on facility policy.	
___	___	___	16. Close the door to the room or pull the bedside curtain.	
___	___	___	17. *Complete necessary assessments before administering medications. Check the patient's allergy bracelet or ask the patient about allergies. Explain the purpose and action of the medication to the patient.*	
___	___	___	18. Scan the patient's bar code on the identification band, if required.	
___	___	___	19. *Based on facility policy, the third check of the label may occur at this point. If so, recheck the labels with the CMAR/MAR before administering the medications to the patient.*	
___	___	___	20. Put on clean gloves.	
___	___	___	21. Select an appropriate administration site.	
___	___	___	22. Assist the patient to the appropriate position for the site chosen. Drape, as needed, to expose only the area of the site to be used.	
___	___	___	23. Identify the appropriate landmarks for the site chosen.	
___	___	___	24. Cleanse the area around the injection site with an antimicrobial swab. Use a firm, circular motion while moving outward from the injection site. Allow the area to dry.	
___	___	___	25. Remove the needle cap with the nondominant hand, pulling it straight off.	
___	___	___	26. Grasp and bunch the area surrounding the injection site or spread the skin taut at the site.	
___	___	___	27. Hold the syringe in the dominant hand between the thumb and forefinger. Inject the needle quickly at a 45- to 90-degree angle.	
___	___	___	28. After the needle is in place, release the tissue. If you have a large skin fold pinched up, ensure that the needle stays in place as the skin is released. Immediately move your nondominant hand to steady the lower end of the syringe. Slide your dominant hand to the end of the plunger. Avoid moving the syringe.	

Excellent	Satisfactory	Needs Practice	SKILL 28-6 **Administering a Subcutaneous Injection** *(Continued)*	Comments
___	___	___	29. Inject the medication slowly (at a rate of 10 sec/mL).	
___	___	___	30. Withdraw the needle quickly at the same angle at which it was inserted, while supporting the surrounding tissue with your nondominant hand.	
___	___	___	31. Using a gauze square, apply gentle pressure to the site after the needle is withdrawn. ***Do not massage the site.***	
___	___	___	32. Do not recap the used needle. Engage the safety shield or needle guard. Discard the needle and syringe in the appropriate receptacle.	
___	___	___	33. Assist the patient to a position of comfort.	
___	___	___	34. Remove gloves and additional PPE, if used. Perform hand hygiene.	
___	___	___	35. Document the administration of the medication immediately after administration.	
___	___	___	36. Evaluate the patient's response to the medication within an appropriate time frame for the particular medication.	

Skill Checklists for Fundamentals of Nursing:
The Art and Science of Person-Centered Nursing Care, 8th edition

Name _____ Date _____

Unit _____ Position _____

Instructor/Evaluator: _____ Position _____

SKILL 28-7

Administering an Intramuscular Injection

Goal: The patient safely receives the medication via the intramuscular route using a Z-track method.

Excellent	Satisfactory	Needs Practice		Comments
—	—	—	1. Gather equipment. Check each medication order against the original order in the medical record according to facility policy. Clarify any inconsistencies. Check the patient's chart for allergies.	
—	—	—	2. Know the actions, special nursing considerations, safe dose ranges, purpose of administration, and adverse effects of the medications to be administered. Consider the appropriateness of the medication for this patient.	
—	—	—	3. Perform hand hygiene.	
—	—	—	4. Move the medication cart to the outside of the patient's room or prepare for administration in the medication area.	
—	—	—	5. Unlock the medication cart or drawer. Enter the pass code and scan employee identification, if required.	
—	—	—	6. *Prepare medications for one patient at a time.*	
—	—	—	7. Read the CMAR/MAR and select the proper medication from unit stock or the patient's medication drawer.	
—	—	—	8. Compare the label with the CMAR/MAR. Check expiration dates and perform calculations, if necessary. Scan the bar code on the package, if required.	
—	—	—	9. If necessary, withdraw medication from an ampule or vial.	
—	—	—	10. *Depending on facility policy, the third check of the label may occur at this point. If so, when all medications for one patient have been prepared, recheck the labels with the CMAR/MAR before taking the medications to the patient.*	
—	—	—	11. Lock the medication cart before leaving it.	
—	—	—	12. Transport medications to the patient's bedside carefully, and keep the medications in sight at all times.	
—	—	—	13. *Ensure that the patient receives the medications at the correct time.*	
—	—	—	14. Perform hand hygiene and put on PPE, if indicated.	

SKILL 28-7
Administering an Intramuscular Injection *(Continued)*

Excellent	Satisfactory	Needs Practice		Comments
___	___	___	15. *Identify the patient. Compare the information with the CMAR/MAR. The patient should be identified using at least two methods:*	
___	___	___	a. Check the name on the patient's identification band.	
___	___	___	b. Check the identification number on the patient's identification band.	
___	___	___	c. Check the birth date on the patient's identification band.	
___	___	___	d. Ask the patient to state name and birth date, based on facility policy.	
___	___	___	16. Close the door to the room or pull the bedside curtain.	
___	___	___	17. *Complete necessary assessments before administering medications. Check the patient's allergy bracelet or ask the patient about allergies. Explain the purpose and action of the medication to the patient.*	
___	___	___	18. Scan the patient's bar code on the identification band, if required.	
___	___	___	19. *Based on facility policy, the third check of the label may occur at this point. If so, recheck the labels with the CMAR/MAR before administering the medications to the patient.*	
___	___	___	20. Put on clean gloves.	
___	___	___	21. Select an appropriate administration site.	
___	___	___	22. Assist the patient to the appropriate position for the site chosen. Drape, as needed, to expose only the area of site being used.	
___	___	___	23. Identify the appropriate landmarks for the site chosen.	
___	___	___	24. Cleanse the area around the injection site with an antimicrobial swab. Use a firm, circular motion while moving outward from the injection site. Allow the area to dry.	
___	___	___	25. Remove the needle cap by pulling it straight off. Hold the syringe in your dominant hand between the thumb and forefinger.	
___	___	___	26. Displace the skin in a Z-track manner. Pull the skin down or to one side about 1 inch (2.5 cm) with your nondominant hand and hold the skin and tissue in this position.	
___	___	___	27. Quickly dart the needle into the tissue so that the needle is perpendicular to the patient's body. This should ensure that the medication is administered using an injection angle between 72 and 90 degrees.	

Administering an Intramuscular Injection *(Continued)*

Excellent	Satisfactory	Needs Practice		Comments
——	——	——	28. As soon as the needle is in place, use the thumb and forefinger of your nondominant hand to hold the lower end of the syringe. Slide your dominant hand to the end of the plunger. Inject the solution slowly (10 sec/mL of medication).	
——	——	——	29. Once the medication has been instilled, wait 10 seconds before withdrawing the needle.	
——	——	——	30. Withdraw the needle smoothly and steadily at the same angle at which it was inserted, supporting tissue around the injection site with your nondominant hand.	
——	——	——	31. Apply gentle pressure at the site with a dry gauze. ***Do not massage the site.***	
——	——	——	32. Do not recap the used needle. Engage the safety shield or needle guard, if present. Discard the needle and syringe in the appropriate receptacle.	
——	——	——	33. Assist the patient to a position of comfort.	
——	——	——	34. Remove gloves and additional PPE, if used. Perform hand hygiene.	
——	——	——	35. Document the administration of the medication immediately after administration.	
——	——	——	36. Evaluate the patient's response to medication within an appropriate time frame. Assess the site, if possible, within 2 to 4 hours after administration.	

Skill Checklists for Fundamentals of Nursing:
The Art and Science of Person-Centered Nursing Care, 8th edition

Name _____   Date _____

Unit _____   Position _____

Instructor/Evaluator: _____   Position _____

Excellent	Satisfactory	Needs Practice	SKILL 28-8 **Administering Medications by Intravenous Bolus or Push Through an Intravenous Infusion** **Goal:** The prescribed medication is given safely to the patient via the intravenous route.	Comments
___	___	___	1. Gather equipment. Check the medication order against the original order in the medical record, according to facility policy. Clarify any inconsistencies. Check the patient's chart for allergies. Verify the compatibility of the medication and IV fluid. Check a drug resource to clarify whether the medication needs to be diluted before administration. Check the administration rate.	
___	___	___	2. Know the actions, special nursing considerations, safe dose ranges, purpose of administration, and adverse effects of the medications to be administered. Consider the appropriateness of the medication for this patient.	
___	___	___	3. Perform hand hygiene.	
___	___	___	4. Move the medication cart to the outside of the patient's room or prepare for administration in the medication area.	
___	___	___	5. Unlock the medication cart or drawer. Enter the pass code and scan employee identification, if required.	
___	___	___	6. *Prepare medication for one patient at a time.*	
___	___	___	7. Read the CMAR/MAR and select the proper medication from unit stock or the patient's medication drawer.	
___	___	___	8. Compare the label with the CMAR/MAR. Check expiration dates and perform calculations, if necessary. Scan the bar code on the package, if required.	
___	___	___	9. If necessary, withdraw medication from an ampule or vial.	
___	___	___	10. *Depending on facility policy, the third check of the label may occur at this point. If so, when all medications for one patient have been prepared, recheck the labels with the CMAR/MAR before taking the medications to the patient.*	
___	___	___	11. Lock the medication cart before leaving it.	
___	___	___	12. Transport medications and equipment to the patient's bedside carefully, and keep the medications in sight at all times.	
___	___	___	13. *Ensure that the patient receives the medications at the correct time.*	

SKILL 28-8

Administering Medications by Intravenous Bolus or Push Through an Intravenous Infusion *(Continued)*

Excellent	Satisfactory	Needs Practice		Comments

			14. Perform hand hygiene and put on PPE, if indicated.	
			15. *Identify the patient. Compare the information with the CMAR/MAR. The patient should be identified using at least two methods*:	
			a. Check the name on the patient's identification band.	
			b. Check the identification number on the patient's identification band.	
			c. Check the birth date on the patient's identification band.	
			d. Ask the patient to state name and birth date, based on facility policy.	
			16. Close the door to the room or pull the bedside curtain.	
			17. Complete necessary assessments before administering medications. Check the patient's allergy bracelet or ask the patient about allergies. Explain the purpose and action of the medication to the patient.	
			18. Scan the patient's bar code on the identification band, if required.	
			19. *Based on facility policy, the third check of the label may occur at this point. If so, recheck the labels with the CMAR/MAR before administering the medications to the patient.*	
			20. *Assess the IV site for presence of inflammation or infiltration.*	
			21. If IV infusion is being administered via an infusion pump, pause the pump.	
			22. Put on clean gloves.	
			23. Select an injection port on the tubing that is closest to the venipuncture site. Clean the port with an antimicrobial swab.	
			24. Uncap the syringe. Steady the port with your nondominant hand while inserting the syringe into the center of the port.	
			25. Move your nondominant hand to the section of IV tubing just above the injection port. Fold the tubing between your fingers.	
			26. Pull back slightly on the plunger just until blood appears in the tubing.	
			27. *Inject the medication at the recommended rate.*	

SKILL 28-8

Administering Medications by Intravenous Bolus or Push Through an Intravenous Infusion *(Continued)*

Excellent	Satisfactory	Needs Practice		Comments
___	___	___	28. Release the tubing. Remove the syringe. Do not recap the used needle, if used. Engage the safety shield or needle guard, if present. Release the tubing and allow the IV fluid to flow. Discard the needle and syringe in the appropriate receptacle.	
___	___	___	29. Check IV fluid infusion rate. Restart the infusion pump, if appropriate.	
___	___	___	30. Remove gloves and additional PPE, if used. Perform hand hygiene.	
___	___	___	31. Document the administration of the medication immediately after administration.	
___	___	___	32. Evaluate the patient's response to the medication within the appropriate time frame.	

Skill Checklists for Fundamentals of Nursing:
The Art and Science of Person-Centered Nursing Care, 8th edition

Name _____ Date _____

Unit _____ Position _____

Instructor/Evaluator: _____ Position _____

Excellent	Satisfactory	Needs Practice	SKILL 28-9 **Administering a Piggyback Intermittent Intravenous Infusion of Medication**	
			Goal: The medication is delivered safely to the patient via the intravenous route using sterile technique.	**Comments**
___	___	___	1. Gather equipment. Check each medication order against the original order in the medical record, according to facility policy. Clarify any inconsistencies. Check the patient's chart for allergies.	
___	___	___	2. Know the actions, special nursing considerations, safe dose ranges, purpose of administration, and adverse effects of the medications to be administered. Consider the appropriateness of the medication for this patient.	
___	___	___	3. Perform hand hygiene.	
___	___	___	4. Move the medication cart to the outside of the patient's room or prepare for administration in the medication area.	
___	___	___	5. Unlock the medication cart or drawer. Enter the pass code and scan employee identification, if required.	
___	___	___	6. *Prepare medications for one patient at a time.*	
___	___	___	7. Read the CMAR/MAR and select the proper medication from unit stock or the patient's medication drawer.	
___	___	___	8. Compare the label with the CMAR/MAR. Check expiration dates. Confirm the prescribed or appropriate infusion rate. Calculate the drip rate if using the gravity system. Scan the bar code on the package, if required.	
___	___	___	9. *Depending on facility policy, the third check of the label may occur at this point. If so, when all medications for one patient have been prepared, recheck the labels with the CMAR/MAR before taking the medications to the patient.*	
___	___	___	10. Lock the medication cart before leaving it.	
___	___	___	11. Transport medications to the patient's bedside carefully, and keep the medications in sight at all times.	
___	___	___	12. *Ensure that the patient receives the medications at the correct time.*	
___	___	___	13. Perform hand hygiene and put on PPE, if indicated.	
___	___	___	14. *Identify the patient. Compare the information with the CMAR/MAR. The patient should be identified using at least two methods:*	

			SKILL 28-9

Administering a Piggyback Intermittent Intravenous Infusion of Medication *(Continued)*

Excellent	Satisfactory	Needs Practice		Comments
——	——	——	a. Check the name on the patient's identification band.	
——	——	——	b. Check the identification number on the patient's identification band.	
——	——	——	c. Check the birth date on the patient's identification band.	
——	——	——	d. Ask the patient to state name and birth date, based on facility policy.	
——	——	——	15. Close the door to the room or pull the bedside curtain.	
——	——	——	16. *Complete necessary assessments before administering medications. Check the patient's allergy bracelet or ask the patient about allergies. Explain the purpose and action of the medication to the patient.*	
——	——	——	17. Scan the patient's bar code on the identification band, if required.	
——	——	——	18. *Based on facility policy, the third check of the label may occur at this point. If so, recheck the labels with the CMAR/MAR before administering the medications to the patient.*	
——	——	——	19. Assess the IV site for the presence of inflammation or infiltration.	
——	——	——	20. Close the clamp on the short secondary infusion tubing. Using aseptic technique, remove the cap on the tubing spike and the cap on the port of the medication container, taking care to avoid contaminating either end.	
——	——	——	21. Attach infusion tubing to the medication container by inserting the tubing spike into the port with a firm push and twisting motion, taking care to avoid contaminating either end.	
——	——	——	22. Hang piggyback container on an IV pole, positioning it higher than the primary IV according to manufacturer's recommendations. Use metal or plastic hook to lower primary IV fluid container.	
——	——	——	23. Place a label on the tubing with the appropriate date.	
——	——	——	24. Squeeze the drip chamber on the tubing and release. Fill to the line, or about half full. Open the clamp and prime the tubing. Close the clamp. Place the needleless connector on the end of the tubing, using sterile technique, if required.	
——	——	——	25. Use an antimicrobial swab to clean the access port or stopcock above the roller clamp on the primary IV infusion tubing.	
——	——	——	26. Connect the piggyback setup to the access port or stopcock. If using, turn the stopcock to the open position.	

Administering a Piggyback Intermittent Intravenous Infusion of Medication *(Continued)*

Excellent	Satisfactory	Needs Practice		Comments
——	——	——	27. Open the clamp on the secondary tubing. Set the rate for the secondary infusion on the infusion pump and begin the infusion. If using gravity infusion, use the roller clamp on the primary infusion tubing to regulate flow at the prescribed delivery rate. Monitor medication infusion at periodic intervals.	
——	——	——	28. Clamp the tubing on the piggyback set when the solution is infused. Follow facility policy regarding disposal of equipment.	
——	——	——	29. Raise primary IV fluid container to its original height. *Check the primary infusion rate on the infusion pump. If using gravity infusion, readjust the flow rate of the primary IV.*	
——	——	——	30. Remove PPE, if used. Perform hand hygiene.	
——	——	——	31. Document the administration of the medication immediately after administration.	
——	——	——	32. Evaluate the patient's response to medication within the appropriate time frame. Monitor the IV site at periodic intervals.	

Skill Checklists for Fundamentals of Nursing:
The Art and Science of Person-Centered Nursing Care, 8th edition

Name _____ Date _____

Unit _____ Position _____

Instructor/Evaluator: _____ Position _____

SKILL 28-10

Introducing Drugs Through a Medication or Drug-Infusion Lock (Intermittent Peripheral Venous Access Device) Using the Saline Flush

Goal: The medication is delivered safely to the patient via the intravenous route using sterile technique.

Excellent	Satisfactory	Needs Practice		Comments
___	___	___	1. Gather equipment. Check the medication order against the original order in the medical record, according to agency policy. Clarify any inconsistencies. Check the patient's chart for allergies. Check a drug resource to clarify whether the medication needs to be diluted before administration. Verify the recommended administration rate.	
___	___	___	2. Know the actions, special nursing considerations, safe dose ranges, purpose of administration, and adverse effects of the medications to be administered. Consider the appropriateness of the medication for this patient.	
___	___	___	3. Perform hand hygiene.	
___	___	___	4. Move the medication cart to the outside of the patient's room or prepare for administration in the medication area.	
___	___	___	5. Unlock the medication cart or drawer. Enter the pass code and scan employee identification, if required.	
___	___	___	6. *Prepare medication for one patient at a time.*	
___	___	___	7. Read the CMAR/MAR and select the proper medication from unit stock or the patient's medication drawer.	
___	___	___	8. Compare the label with the CMAR/MAR. Check expiration dates and perform calculations, if necessary. Scan the bar code on the package, if required.	
___	___	___	9. If necessary, withdraw the medication from an ampule or vial.	
___	___	___	10. *Depending on facility policy, the third check of the label may occur at this point. If so, when all medications for one patient have been prepared, recheck the labels with the CMAR/MAR before taking the medications to the patient.*	
___	___	___	11. Lock the medication cart before leaving it.	
___	___	___	12. Transport medications and equipment to the patient's bedside carefully, and keep the medications in sight at all times.	
___	___	___	13. *Ensure that the patient receives the medications at the correct time.*	

Excellent	Satisfactory	Needs Practice		

SKILL 28-10

Introducing Drugs Through a Medication or Drug-Infusion Lock (Intermittent Peripheral Venous Access Device) Using the Saline Flush (Continued)

Comments

Excellent	Satisfactory	Needs Practice	Step	Comments
___	___	___	14. Perform hand hygiene and put on PPE, if indicated.	
___	___	___	15. *Identify the patient. Compare the information with the CMAR/MAR. The patient should be identified using at least two methods:*	
___	___	___	a. Check the name on the patient's identification band.	
___	___	___	b. Check the identification number on the patient's identification band.	
___	___	___	c. Check the birth date on the patient's identification band.	
___	___	___	d. Ask the patient to state name and birth date, based on facility policy.	
___	___	___	16. Close the door to the room or pull the bedside curtain.	
___	___	___	17. *Complete necessary assessments before administering medications. Check the patient's allergy bracelet or ask the patient about allergies. Explain the purpose and action of the medication to the patient.*	
___	___	___	18. Scan the patient's bar code on the identification band, if required.	
___	___	___	19. *Based on facility policy, the third check of the label may occur at this point. If so, recheck the labels with the CMAR/MAR before administering the medications to the patient.*	
___	___	___	20. Assess the IV site for the presence of inflammation or infiltration.	
___	___	___	21. Put on clean gloves.	
___	___	___	22. Clean the access port of the medication lock with an antimicrobial swab.	
___	___	___	23. Stabilize the port with your nondominant hand and insert the syringe, or needleless access device, of normal saline into the access port.	
___	___	___	24. Release the clamp on the extension tubing of the medication lock. Aspirate gently and check for blood return.	
___	___	___	25. Gently flush with normal saline by pushing slowly on the syringe plunger. Observe the insertion site while inserting the saline. Remove the syringe.	
___	___	___	26. Insert the syringe, or needleless access device, with the medication into the port and gently inject the medication, using a watch to verify correct administration rate. *Do not force the injection if resistance is felt.*	

SKILL 28-10

Introducing Drugs Through a Medication or Drug-Infusion Lock (Intermittent Peripheral Venous Access Device) Using the Saline Flush *(Continued)*

Excellent	Satisfactory	Needs Practice		Comments
——	——	——	27. Remove the medication syringe from the port. Stabilize the port with your nondominant hand and insert the syringe, or needleless access device, of normal saline into the port. Gently flush with normal saline by pushing slowly on the syringe plunger. If the medication lock is capped with a positive pressure valve/device, remove the syringe, then clamp the extension tubing. Alternately, to gain positive pressure if a positive pressure valve/device is not present, clamp the extension tubing as you are still flushing the last of the saline into the medication lock. Remove the syringe.	
——	——	——	28. Discard the syringe in the appropriate receptacle.	
——	——	——	29. Remove PPE, if used. Perform hand hygiene.	
——	——	——	30. Document the administration of the medication immediately after administration.	
——	——	——	31. Evaluate the patient's response to the medication within the appropriate time frame.	
——	——	——	32. Check the medication lock site at least every 8 hours or according to facility policy.	

Skill Checklists for Fundamentals of Nursing:
The Art and Science of Person-Centered Nursing Care, 8th edition

Name _____ Date _____

Unit _____ Position _____

Instructor/Evaluator: _____ Position _____

SKILL 29-1

Providing Preoperative Patient Care: Hospitalized Patient

Goal: The patient will be prepared physically and psychologically to proceed to surgery.

Excellent	Satisfactory	Needs Practice		Comments
——	——	——	1. Check the patient's medical record for the type of surgery and review the medical orders. Review the nursing database, history, and physical examination. Check that the baseline data are recorded; report those that are abnormal.	
——	——	——	2. *Check that all diagnostic testing has been completed and results are available; identify and report abnormal results.* Gather the necessary supplies.	
——	——	——	3. Perform hand hygiene and put on PPE, if indicated.	
——	——	——	4. Identify the patient.	
——	——	——	5. Close the curtains around the bed and close the door to the room, if possible. Explain to the patient and significant other what you are going to do and why you are going to do it. Place necessary supplies on the bedside stand or overbed table, within easy reach.	
——	——	——	6. Explore the psychological needs of the patient and family related to the surgery.	
——	——	——	a. Establish a therapeutic relationship, encouraging the patient to verbalize concerns or fears.	
——	——	——	b. Use active listening skills, answering questions and clarifying any misinformation.	
——	——	——	c. Use touch, as appropriate, to convey genuine empathy.	
——	——	——	d. Offer to contact spiritual counselor (e.g., priest, minister, rabbi) to meet spiritual needs.	
——	——	——	7. *Identify learning needs of the patient and family.* Ensure that the informed consent of the patient for the surgery has been signed, timed, dated, and witnessed. Inquire if the patient has any questions regarding the surgical procedure. Check the patient's record to determine if an advance directive has been completed. If an advance directive has not been completed, discuss with the patient the possibility of completing it, as appropriate. If the patient has had surgery before, ask about this experience.	
——	——	——	8. Teach deep breathing exercises.	
——	——	——	9. Teach coughing and splinting.	

Excellent	Satisfactory	Needs Practice		Comments
			SKILL 29-1 **Providing Preoperative Patient Care:** **Hospitalized Patient** *(Continued)*	
___	___	___	10. Teach use of incentive spirometer.	
___	___	___	11. Teach leg exercises, as appropriate.	
___	___	___	12. Assist the patient in putting on graduated compression stockings and demonstrate how the pneumatic compression device operates.	
___	___	___	13. Teach turning in the bed.	
___	___	___	a. Instruct the patient to use a pillow or bath blanket to splint where the incision will be. Ask the patient to raise the left knee and reach across to grasp the right side rail of the bed when turning toward the patient's right side. If turning to the left side, the patient will bend the right knee and grasp the left side rail.	
___	___	___	b. When turning the patient onto the right side, ask the patient to push with bent left leg and pull on the right side rail. Explain that you will place a pillow behind the patient's back to provide support, and that the call bell will be placed within easy reach.	
___	___	___	c. Explain to the patient that position change is recommended every 2 hours.	
___	___	___	14. Teach pain management.	
___	___	___	a. Discuss past experiences with pain and interventions that the patient has used to reduce pain.	
___	___	___	b. Discuss the availability of analgesic medication postoperatively.	
___	___	___	c. Discuss the use of patient-controlled analgesia (PCA), as appropriate.	
___	___	___	d. Explore the use of other alternative and nonpharmacologic methods to reduce pain, such as position change, massage, relaxation/diversion, guided imagery, and meditation.	
___	___	___	15. Review equipment that may be used after surgery.	
___	___	___	a. Show the patient various types of equipment, such as IV pumps, electronic blood pressure cuff, tubes, and surgical drains.	
___	___	___	16. Provide skin preparation.	
___	___	___	a. *Ask the patient to bathe or shower with the antiseptic solution. Remind the patient to clean the surgical site.*	
___	___	___	17. Provide teaching about and follow dietary/fluid restrictions. *Explain to the patient that both food and fluid will be restricted before surgery to ensure that the stomach contains a minimal amount of gastric secretions. This*	

Excellent	Satisfactory	Needs Practice	SKILL 29-1 **Providing Preoperative Patient Care: Hospitalized Patient** *(Continued)*	
				Comments
			restriction is important to reduce the risk of aspiration. Emphasize to the patient the importance of avoiding food and fluids during the prescribed time period, because failure to adhere may necessitate cancellation of the surgery.	
——	——	——	18. Provide intestinal preparation, as appropriate. In certain situations, the bowel will need to be prepared by administering enemas or laxatives to evacuate the bowel and to reduce the intestinal bacteria.	
——	——	——	a. As needed, provide explanation of the purpose of enemas or laxatives before surgery. If patient will be administering an enema, clarify the steps as needed.	
——	——	——	19. *Check administration of regularly scheduled medications.* Review with the patient routine medications, over-the-counter medications, and herbal supplements that are taken regularly. Check the medical orders and review with the patient which medications will be permitted the day of surgery.	
——	——	——	20. Remove PPE, if used. Perform hand hygiene.	

Skill Checklists for Fundamentals of Nursing:
The Art and Science of Person-Centered Nursing Care, 8th edition

Name _____   Date _____

Unit _____   Position _____

Instructor/Evaluator: _____   Position _____

Excellent	Satisfactory	Needs Practice	SKILL 29-2 **Providing Postoperative Care When Patient Returns to Room**	
			Goal: The patient will recover from the surgery with postoperative risks minimized by frequent assessments.	**Comments**
			Immediate Care	
____	____	____	1. When patient returns from the PACU, participate in hand-off report from the PACU nurse and review the operating room and PACU data. Gather the necessary supplies.	
____	____	____	2. Perform hand hygiene and put on PPE, if indicated.	
____	____	____	3. Identify the patient.	
____	____	____	4. Close the curtains around the bed and close the door to the room, if possible. Explain to the patient or significant other what you are going to do and why you are going to do it. Place necessary supplies on the bedside stand or overbed table, within easy reach.	
____	____	____	5. *Place patient in safe position (semi- or high Fowler's or side-lying). Note level of consciousness.*	
____	____	____	6. *Obtain vital signs. Monitor and record vital signs frequently.* Assessment order may vary, but usual frequency includes taking vital signs every 15 minutes the first hour, every 30 minutes the next 2 hours, every hour for 4 hours, and finally every 4 hours.	
____	____	____	7. Assess the patient's respiratory status. Measure the patient's oxygen saturation level.	
____	____	____	8. Assess the patient's cardiovascular status.	
____	____	____	9. Assess the patient's neurovascular status, based on the type of surgery performed.	
____	____	____	10. Provide for warmth, using heated or extra blankets, as necessary. Assess skin color and condition.	
____	____	____	11. Check dressings for color, odor, presence of drains, and amount of drainage. Mark the drainage on the dressing by circling the amount, and include the time. Turn the patient to assess visually under the patient for bleeding from the surgical site.	
____	____	____	12. Verify that all tubes and drains are patent and equipment is working; note amount of drainage in collection device. If an indwelling urinary (Foley) catheter is in place, note urinary output.	

SKILL 29-2

Providing Postoperative Care
When Patient Returns to Room *(Continued)*

Excellent	Satisfactory	Needs Practice		Comments
——	——	——	13. Verify and maintain IV infusion at prescribed rate.	
——	——	——	14. Assess for pain and relieve it by administering medications ordered by the primary care provider. If the patient has been instructed in use of PCA for pain management, review its use. Check record to verify if analgesic medication was administered in the PACU.	
——	——	——	15. Provide for a safe environment. Keep bed in low position with side rails up, based on facility policy. Have call bell within patient's reach.	
——	——	——	16. Remove PPE, if used. Perform hand hygiene.	
			Ongoing Care	
——	——	——	17. Promote optimal respiratory function.	
——	——	——	a. Assess respiratory rate, depth, quality, color, and capillary refill. Ask if the patient is experiencing any difficulty breathing.	
——	——	——	b. Assist with coughing and deep breathing exercises.	
——	——	——	c. Assist with incentive spirometry.	
——	——	——	d. Assist with early ambulation.	
——	——	——	e. Provide frequent position changes.	
——	——	——	f. Administer oxygen as ordered.	
——	——	——	g. Monitor pulse oximetry.	
——	——	——	18. Promote optimal cardiovascular function:	
——	——	——	a. Assess apical rate, rhythm, and quality, and compare with peripheral pulses, color, and blood pressure. Ask if the patient has any chest pains or shortness of breath.	
——	——	——	b. Provide frequent position changes.	
——	——	——	c. Assist with early ambulation.	
——	——	——	d. Apply graduated compression stockings or pneumatic compression devices, if ordered and not in place. If in place, assess for integrity.	
——	——	——	e. Provide leg and range-of-motion exercises if not contraindicated.	
——	——	——	19. Promote optimal neurologic function:	
——	——	——	a. Assess level of consciousness, movement, and sensation.	
——	——	——	b. Determine the level of orientation to person, place, and time.	

Excellent	Satisfactory	Needs Practice	

Providing Postoperative Care
When Patient Returns to Room (Continued)

Comments

——	——	——	c. Test motor ability by asking the patient to move each extremity.
——	——	——	d. Evaluate sensation by asking the patient if your touch can be felt on the patient's extremity.
——	——	——	20. Promote optimal renal and urinary function as well as fluid and electrolyte status. Assess intake and output, evaluate for urinary retention, and monitor serum electrolyte levels.
——	——	——	a. Promote voiding by offering bedpan at regular intervals, noting the frequency, amount, and if there are any burning or urgency symptoms.
——	——	——	b. Monitor urinary catheter drainage if present.
——	——	——	c. Measure intake and output.
——	——	——	21. Promote optimal gastrointestinal function and meet nutritional needs:
——	——	——	a. Assess abdomen for distention and firmness. Ask if patient feels nauseated, had been vomiting, and if passing flatus.
——	——	——	b. Auscultate for bowel sounds.
——	——	——	c. Assist with diet progression; encourage fluid intake; monitor intake.
——	——	——	d. Medicate for nausea and vomiting, as ordered.
——	——	——	22. Promote optimal wound healing.
——	——	——	a. Assess condition of wound for presence of drains and any drainage.
——	——	——	b. Use surgical asepsis for dressing changes and drain care.
——	——	——	c. Inspect all skin surfaces for beginning signs of pressure ulcer development and use pressure-relieving supports to minimize potential skin breakdown.
——	——	——	23. Promote optimal comfort and relief from pain.
——	——	——	a. Assess for pain (location and intensity, using pain scale).
——	——	——	b. Provide for rest and comfort; provide extra blankets, as needed, for warmth.
——	——	——	c. Administer pain medications, as needed, and/or initiate nonpharmacologic methods, as appropriate.
——	——	——	24. Promote optimal meeting of psychosocial needs:
——	——	——	a. Provide emotional support to patient and family, as needed.
——	——	——	b. Explain procedures and offer explanations regarding postoperative recovery, as needed, to both patient and family members.

Skill Checklists for Fundamentals of Nursing:
The Art and Science of Person-Centered Nursing Care, 8th edition

Name _____ Date _____

Unit _____ Position _____

Instructor/Evaluator: _____ Position _____

SKILL 30-1

Providing a Bed Bath

Excellent	Satisfactory	Needs Practice		Comments
			Goal: The patient will vocalize feeling clean and fresh.	
——	——	——	1. Review the patient's health record for any limitations in physical activity.	
——	——	——	2. Perform hand hygiene and put on gloves and/or other PPE, if indicated.	
——	——	——	3. Identify the patient. Discuss the procedure with the patient and assess the patient's ability to assist in the bathing process, as well as personal hygiene preferences.	
——	——	——	4. Assemble equipment on overbed table within reach.	
——	——	——	5. Close the curtains around the bed and close the door to the room, if possible. Adjust the room temperature, if necessary.	
——	——	——	6. Adjust the bed to a comfortable working height; usually elbow height of the caregiver.	
——	——	——	7. Remove sequential compression devices and antiembolism stockings from lower extremities according to agency protocol.	
——	——	——	8. Put on gloves. Offer the patient a bedpan or urinal.	
——	——	——	9. Remove gloves and perform hand hygiene.	
——	——	——	10. Put on a clean pair of gloves. Lower the side rail nearer to you and assist the patient to the side of bed where you will work. Have the patient lie on his or her back.	
——	——	——	11. Loosen top covers and remove all except the top sheet. Place the bath blanket over the patient, then remove the top sheet while the patient holds the bath blanket in place. If the linen is to be reused, fold it over a chair. Place soiled linen in a laundry bag. Take care to prevent the linen from coming in contact with your clothing.	
——	——	——	12. Remove the patient's gown and keep the bath blanket in place. If the patient has an IV line and is not wearing a gown with snap sleeves, remove the gown from the other arm first. Lower the IV container and pass the gown over the tubing and the container. *Rehang the container and check the drip rate.*	

Excellent	Satisfactory	Needs Practice	SKILL 30-1 **Providing a Bed Bath** (Continued)	Comments
——	——	——	13. *Raise side rails.* Fill the basin with a sufficient amount of comfortably warm water (100°F to 120°F to 125°F). Add skin cleanser, if appropriate, according to the manufacturer's directions. Change as necessary throughout the bath. Lower the side rail closer to you when you return to the bedside to begin the bath.	
——	——	——	14. Put on gloves, if necessary. If desired, fold the washcloth like a mitt on your hand so that there are no loose ends.	
——	——	——	15. Lay a towel across the patient's chest and on top of the bath blanket.	
——	——	——	16. *With no cleanser on the washcloth, wipe one eye from the inner part of the eye, near the nose, to the outer part. Rinse or turn the cloth before washing the other eye.*	
——	——	——	17. Bathe the patient's face, neck, and ears. Apply appropriate emollient.	
——	——	——	18. Expose the patient's far arm and place the towel lengthwise under it. Using firm strokes, wash the hand, arm, and axilla, lifting the arm as necessary to access axillary region. Rinse, if necessary, and dry. Apply an appropriate emollient.	
——	——	——	19. Place a folded towel on the bed next to the patient's hand and put the basin on it. Soak the patient's hand in the basin. Wash, rinse if necessary, and dry the hand. Apply an appropriate emollient.	
——	——	——	20. Repeat Actions 18 and 19 for the arm nearer you. An option for the nurse who is shorter or susceptible to back strain might be to bathe one side of the patient first, then move to the other side of the bed to complete the bath.	
——	——	——	21. Spread a towel across the patient's chest. Lower the bath blanket to the patient's umbilical area. Wash, rinse, if necessary, and dry the chest. Keep the chest covered with the towel between the wash and rinse. Pay special attention to the folds of skin under the breasts. Apply an appropriate emollient.	
——	——	——	22. Lower the bath blanket to the perineal area. Place a towel over the patient's chest.	
——	——	——	23. Wash, rinse, if necessary, and dry abdomen. Carefully inspect and clean umbilical area and any abdominal folds or creases. Apply an appropriate emollient.	
——	——	——	24. Return the bath blanket to its original position and expose the far leg. Place the towel under the far leg. Using firm strokes, wash, rinse if necessary, and dry the leg from the ankle to the knee and the knee to the groin. Apply an appropriate emollient.	

SKILL 30-1
Providing a Bed Bath *(Continued)*

Excellent	Satisfactory	Needs Practice		Comments
——	——	——	25. Wash, rinse if necessary, and dry the foot. Pay particular attention to the areas between the toes. Apply an appropriate emollient.	
——	——	——	26. Repeat Actions 24 and 25 for the other leg and foot.	
——	——	——	27. Make sure the patient is covered with the bath blanket. Change the water and washcloth at this point or earlier, if necessary.	
——	——	——	28. Assist the patient to a prone or side-lying position. Put on gloves, if not applied earlier. Position the bath blanket and towel to expose only the back and buttocks.	
——	——	——	29. Wash, rinse if necessary, and dry back and buttocks area. *Pay particular attention to cleansing between the gluteal folds, and observe for any redness or skin breakdown in the sacral area.*	
——	——	——	30. If not contraindicated, give patient a backrub. Alternatively, a back massage may be given after perineal care. Apply an appropriate emollient and/or skin barrier product.	
——	——	——	31. Raise the side rail. Refill the basin with clean water. Discard the washcloth and towel. Remove gloves and put on clean gloves.	
——	——	——	32. Clean the perineal area or set the patient up to allow the patient to complete perineal self-care. If the patient is unable, lower the side rail and complete perineal care. Apply skin barrier, as indicated. Raise the side rail, remove gloves, and perform hand hygiene.	
——	——	——	33. Help the patient put on a clean gown and assist with the use of other personal toiletries, such as deodorant or cosmetics.	
——	——	——	34. Protect the pillow with a towel and groom the patient's hair.	
——	——	——	35. *When finished, make sure that the patient is comfortable, with the side rails up and the bed in the lowest position.*	
——	——	——	36. Change the bed linens. Dispose of soiled linens according to facility policy. Clean the bath basin according to facility policy before returning it to storage at the bedside. Remove gloves and any other PPE, if used. Perform hand hygiene.	

Skill Checklists for Fundamentals of Nursing:
The Art and Science of Person-Centered Nursing Care, 8th edition

Name _____ Date _____

Unit _____ Position _____

Instructor/Evaluator: _____ Position _____

SKILL 30-2
Assisting the Patient With Oral Care

Goal: The patient will have a clean mouth and clean teeth, exhibit a positive body image, and verbalize the importance of oral care.

Excellent	Satisfactory	Needs Practice		Comments
___	___	___	1. Perform hand hygiene and put on gloves if assisting with oral care, and/or other PPE, if indicated.	
___	___	___	2. Identify the patient. Explain the procedure to the patient.	
___	___	___	3. Assemble equipment on the overbed table within the patient's reach.	
___	___	___	4. Close the room door or curtains. Place the bed at an appropriate and comfortable working height, usually elbow height of the caregiver.	
___	___	___	5. Lower the side rail and assist the patient to a sitting position, if permitted, or turn the patient onto the side. Place the towel across the patient's chest.	
___	___	___	6. Encourage the patient to brush own teeth according to the following guidelines. Assist, if necessary.	
___	___	___	a. Moisten the toothbrush and apply toothpaste to the bristles.	
___	___	___	b. Place the brush at a 45-degree angle to the gum line and brush from the gum line to the crown of each tooth. Brush the outer and inner surfaces. Brush back and forth across the biting surface of each tooth.	
___	___	___	c. Brush the tongue gently with the toothbrush.	
___	___	___	d. Have the patient rinse vigorously with water and spit into the emesis basin. Repeat until clear. Suction may be used as an alternative for removal of fluid and secretions from the mouth.	
___	___	___	7. Assist the patient to floss teeth, if appropriate:	
___	___	___	a. Remove approximately 6 inches of dental floss from the container or use a plastic floss holder. Wrap the floss around the index fingers, keeping about 1 to 1.5 inches of floss taut between the fingers.	
___	___	___	b. Insert the floss gently between the teeth, moving it back and forth downward to the gums.	

Assisting the Patient With Oral Care *(Continued)*

Excellent	Satisfactory	Needs Practice		Comments
——	——	——	c. Move the floss up and down, first on one side of a tooth and then on the other side of the tooth, until the surfaces are clean. Repeat in the spaces between all teeth.	
——	——	——	d. Instruct the patient to rinse the mouth well with water after flossing.	
——	——	——	8. Offer mouthwash if the patient prefers.	
——	——	——	9. Offer lip balm or petroleum jelly.	
——	——	——	10. Remove equipment. Remove gloves and discard. Raise the side rail and lower the bed. Assist the patient to a position of comfort.	
——	——	——	11. Remove any other PPE, if used. Perform hand hygiene.	

Name _____   Date _____

Unit _____   Position _____

Instructor/Evaluator: _____   Position _____

SKILL 30-3
Providing Oral Care for the Dependent Patient

Excellent	Satisfactory	Needs Practice	**Goal:** The patient's mouth and teeth will be clean; the patient will not experience impaired oral mucous membranes; the patient will demonstrate improvement in body image; and the patient will verbalize, if able, an understanding about the importance of oral care.	Comments
___	___	___	1. Perform hand hygiene and put on PPE, if indicated.	
___	___	___	2. Identify the patient. Explain the procedure to the patient.	
___	___	___	3. Assemble equipment on the overbed table within reach.	
___	___	___	4. Close the room door or curtains. Place the bed at an appropriate and comfortable working height, usually elbow height of the caregiver. Lower one side rail and position the patient on the side, with the head tilted forward. Place the towel across the patient's chest and the emesis basin in position under the chin. Put on gloves.	
___	___	___	5. Gently open the patient's mouth by applying pressure to the lower jaw at the front of the mouth. Remove dentures, if present. Brush the teeth and gums carefully with a toothbrush and paste. Lightly brush the tongue.	
___	___	___	6. Use a Toothette dipped in water to rinse the oral cavity. If desired, insert the rubber tip of the irrigating syringe into the patient's mouth and rinse gently with a small amount of water. *Position the patient's head to allow for return of water or use the suction apparatus to remove the water from the oral cavity.*	
___	___	___	7. Clean the dentures before replacing.	
___	___	___	8. Apply lubricant to the patient's lips.	
___	___	___	9. Remove equipment and return the patient to a position of comfort. Remove your gloves. Raise the side rail and lower the bed.	
___	___	___	10. Remove additional PPE, if used. Perform hand hygiene.	

Skill Checklists for Fundamentals of Nursing:
The Art and Science of Person-Centered Nursing Care, 8th edition

Name _____ Date _____

Unit _____ Position _____

Instructor/Evaluator: _____ Position _____

Excellent	Satisfactory	Needs Practice	SKILL 30-4 **Making an Unoccupied Bed**	Comments
			Goal: The bed linens will be changed without injury to the nurse or patient.	
___	___	___	1. Perform hand hygiene. Put on PPE, as indicated.	
___	___	___	2. Explain to the patient what you are going to do and the reason for doing it, if the patient is present in the room.	
___	___	___	3. Assemble necessary equipment on the bedside stand or overbed table.	
___	___	___	4. Adjust the bed to a comfortable working height, usually elbow height of the caregiver. Drop the side rails.	
___	___	___	5. Disconnect call bell or any tubes from bed linens.	
___	___	___	6. Put on gloves. Loosen all linen as you move around the bed, from the head of the bed on the far side to the head of the bed on the near side.	
___	___	___	7. Fold reusable linens, such as sheets, blankets, or spread, in place on the bed in fourths and hang them over a clean chair.	
___	___	___	8. Snugly roll all the soiled linen inside the bottom sheet and place directly into the laundry hamper. *Do not place on the floor or furniture. Do not hold soiled linens against your uniform.*	
___	___	___	9. If possible, shift the mattress up to the head of bed. If the mattress is soiled, clean and dry according to facility policy before applying new sheets.	
___	___	___	10. Remove your gloves, unless indicated for transmission-based precautions. Place the bottom sheet with its center fold in the center of the bed. Open the sheet and fan-fold to the center.	
___	___	___	11. Pull the bottom sheet over the corners at the head and foot of the mattress.	

Excellent	Satisfactory	Needs Practice	SKILL 30-5 **Making an Occupied Bed** (Continued)	
				Comments
——	——	——	15. If using, place the drawsheet with its center fold in the center of the bed and positioned so that it will be located under the patient's midsection. Open the drawsheet and fan-fold to the center of the mattress. Tuck the drawsheet securely under the mattress. If a protective pad is used, place it over the drawsheet in the proper area and open to the center fold. Not all facilities use drawsheets routinely. The nurse may decide to use one.	
——	——	——	16. Raise the side rail. Assist the patient to roll over the folded linen in the middle of the bed toward you. Reposition the pillow and bath blanket or top sheet. Move to the other side of the bed and lower the side rail.	
——	——	——	17. Loosen and remove all bottom linen. Discard soiled linen in the laundry bag or hamper. ***Do not place on the floor or furniture. Do not hold soiled linens against your uniform.***	
——	——	——	18. Ease clean linen from under the patient. Pull the bottom sheet taut and secure at the corners at the head and foot of the mattress. Pull the drawsheet tight and smooth. Tuck the drawsheet securely under the mattress.	
——	——	——	19. Assist the patient to turn back to the center of bed. Remove the pillow and change the pillowcase. Open each pillowcase in the same manner as you opened the other linens. Gather the pillowcase over one hand toward the closed end. Grasp the pillow with the hand inside the pillowcase. Keep a firm hold on the top of the pillow and pull the cover onto the pillow. Place the pillow under the patient's head.	
——	——	——	20. Apply the top linens, sheet and blanket, if desired, so that it is centered. Fold the top linens over at the patient's shoulders to make a cuff. Have the patient hold on to the top linens and remove the bath blanket from underneath.	
——	——	——	21. Secure top linens under the foot of the mattress and miter corners. Loosen the top linens over the patient's feet by grasping them in the area of the feet and pulling gently toward the foot of the bed.	
——	——	——	22. Return the patient to a position of comfort. Remove your gloves. Raise the side rail and lower the bed. Reattach the call bell.	
——	——	——	23. Dispose of soiled linens according to agency policy.	
——	——	——	24. Remove any other PPE, if used. Perform hand hygiene.	

Skill Checklists for Fundamentals of Nursing:
The Art and Science of Person-Centered Nursing Care, 8th edition

Name _____   Date _____

Unit _____   Position _____

Instructor/Evaluator: _____   Position _____

SKILL 31-1

Cleaning a Wound and Applying a Dry, Sterile Dressing

Goal: The wound is cleaned and protected with a dressing without contaminating the wound area, without causing trauma to the wound, and without causing the patient to experience pain or discomfort.

Excellent	Satisfactory	Needs Practice		Comments
——	——	——	1. Review the medical order for wound care or the nursing plan of care related to wound care. Gather necessary supplies.	
——	——	——	2. Perform hand hygiene and put on PPE, if indicated.	
——	——	——	3. Identify the patient.	
——	——	——	4. Assemble equipment on the overbed table within reach.	
——	——	——	5. Close curtains around the bed and close the door to the room if possible. Explain to the patient what you are going to do and why you are going to do it.	
——	——	——	6. Assess the patient for the possible need for nonpharmacologic pain-reducing interventions or analgesic medication before wound care dressing change. Administer appropriate prescribed analgesic. Allow enough time for the analgesic to achieve its effectiveness.	
——	——	——	7. Place a waste receptacle or bag at a convenient location for use during the procedure.	
——	——	——	8. Adjust the bed to a comfortable working height, usually elbow height of the caregiver.	
——	——	——	9. Assist the patient to a comfortable position that provides easy access to the wound area. Use the bath blanket to cover any exposed area other than the wound. Place a waterproof pad under the wound site.	
——	——	——	10. Check the position of drains, tubes, or other adjuncts before removing the dressing. Put on clean, disposable gloves and loosen tape on the old dressings. If necessary, use an adhesive remover to help get the tape off.	
——	——	——	11. Carefully remove the soiled dressings. If there is resistance, use a silicone-based adhesive remover to help remove the tape. If any part of the dressing sticks to the underlying skin, use small amounts of sterile saline to help loosen and remove it.	

Excellent	Satisfactory	Needs Practice	SKILL 31-1 **Cleaning a Wound and Applying a Dry, Sterile Dressing** *(Continued)*	
				Comments
——	——	——	12. After removing the dressing, note the presence, amount, type, color, and odor of any drainage on the dressings. Place soiled dressings in the appropriate waste receptacle. Remove your gloves and dispose of them in an appropriate waste receptacle.	
——	——	——	13. Inspect the wound site for size, appearance, and drainage. Assess if any pain is present. Check the status of sutures, adhesive closure strips, staples, and drains or tubes, if present. Note any problems to include in your documentation.	
——	——	——	14. *Using sterile technique, prepare a sterile work area and open the needed supplies.*	
——	——	——	15. Open the sterile cleaning solution. Depending on the amount of cleaning needed, the solution might be poured directly over gauze sponges over a container for small cleaning jobs, or into a basin for more complex or larger cleaning.	
——	——	——	16. Put on sterile gloves. Alternately, clean gloves (clean technique) may be used when cleaning a chronic wound or pressure ulcer.	
——	——	——	17. Clean the wound. *Clean the wound from top to bottom and from the center to the outside.* Following this pattern, use new gauze for each wipe, placing the used gauze in the waste receptacle. Alternately, spray the wound from top to bottom with a commercially prepared wound cleanser.	
——	——	——	18. Once the wound is cleaned, dry the area using a gauze sponge in the same manner. Apply ointment or perform other treatments, as ordered.	
——	——	——	19. If a drain is in use at the wound location, clean around the drain.	
——	——	——	20. Apply a layer of dry, sterile dressing over the wound. Forceps may be used to apply the dressing.	
——	——	——	21. Place a second layer of gauze over the wound site, as necessary.	
——	——	——	22. Apply a surgical or abdominal pad (ABD) over the gauze at the site as the outermost layer of the dressing, as necessary.	
——	——	——	23. Remove and discard gloves. Apply tape, Montgomery straps or roller gauze to secure the dressings. Alternately, many commercial wound products are self-adhesive and do not require additional tape.	

SKILL 31-1

Cleaning a Wound and Applying a Dry, Sterile Dressing *(Continued)*

Excellent	Satisfactory	Needs Practice		Comments
——	——	——	24. After securing the dressing, label it with date and time. Remove all remaining equipment; place the patient in a comfortable position, with the side rails up and the bed in the lowest position.	
——	——	——	25. Remove PPE, if used. Perform hand hygiene.	
——	——	——	26. Check all wound dressings every shift. More frequent checks may be needed if the wound is more complex or dressings become saturated quickly.	

Skill Checklists for Fundamentals of Nursing:
The Art and Science of Person-Centered Nursing Care, 8th edition

Name _____   Date _____

Unit _____   Position _____

Instructor/Evaluator: _____   Position _____

SKILL 31-2

Applying a Saline-Moistened Dressing

Excellent	Satisfactory	Needs Practice		Comments
			Goal: The procedure is accomplished without contaminating the wound area, without causing trauma to the wound, and without causing the patient to experience pain or discomfort.	
___	___	___	1. Review the medical orders for wound care or the nursing plan of care related to wound care. Gather necessary supplies.	
___	___	___	2. Perform hand hygiene and put on PPE, if indicated.	
___	___	___	3. Identify the patient.	
___	___	___	4. Assemble equipment on the overbed table within reach.	
___	___	___	5. Close the curtains around the bed and close the door to the room if possible. Explain what you are going to do and why you are going to do it to the patient.	
			6. Assess the patient for possible need for nonpharmacologic pain-reducing interventions or analgesic medication before wound care dressing change. Administer the appropriate prescribed analgesic. Allow enough time for the analgesic to achieve its effectiveness.	
___	___	___	7. Place a waste receptacle or bag at a convenient location for use during the procedure.	
___	___	___	8. Adjust the bed to a comfortable working height, usually elbow height of the caregiver.	
			9. Assist the patient to a comfortable position that provides easy access to the wound area. Position the patient so that the wound cleanser or irrigation solution will flow from the clean end of the wound toward the dirtier end, if being used. Use the bath blanket to cover any exposed area other than the wound. Place a waterproof pad under the wound site.	
___	___	___	10. Put on clean gloves. Carefully and gently remove the soiled dressings. If there is resistance, use a silicone-based adhesive remover to help remove the tape. If any part of the dressing sticks to the underlying skin, use small amounts of sterile saline to help loosen and remove it.	
___	___	___	11. After removing the dressing, note the presence, amount, type, color, and odor of any drainage on the dressings. Place soiled dressings in the appropriate waste receptacle.	

SKILL 31-2

Applying a Saline-Moistened Dressing *(Continued)*

Excellent	Satisfactory	Needs Practice		Comments
——	——	——	12. Assess the wound for appearance, stage, the presence of eschar, granulation tissue, epithelialization, undermining, tunneling, necrosis, sinus tract, and drainage. Assess the appearance of the surrounding tissue. Measure the wound.	
——	——	——	13. Remove your gloves and put them in the receptacle.	
——	——	——	14. Using sterile technique, open the supplies and dressings. Place the fine-mesh gauze into the basin and pour the ordered solution over the mesh to saturate it.	
——	——	——	15. Put on sterile gloves. Alternately, clean gloves (clean technique) may be used to clean a chronic wound or pressure ulcer.	
——	——	——	16. Clean the wound. Alternately, irrigate the wound, as ordered or required.	
——	——	——	17. Dry the surrounding skin with sterile gauze dressings.	
——	——	——	18. Apply a skin protectant to the surrounding skin, if needed.	
——	——	——	19. If not already on, put on sterile gloves. Squeeze excess fluid from the gauze dressing. Unfold and fluff the dressing.	
——	——	——	20. Gently press to loosely pack the moistened gauze into the wound. If necessary, use the forceps or cotton-tipped applicators to press the gauze into all wound surfaces.	
——	——	——	21. Apply several dry, sterile gauze pads over the wet gauze.	
——	——	——	22. Place the ABD pad over the gauze.	
——	——	——	23. Remove and discard gloves. Apply tape, Montgomery straps or roller gauze to secure the dressings. Alternately, many commercial wound products are self-adhesive and do not require additional tape.	
——	——	——	24. After securing the dressing, label the dressing with the date and time. Remove all remaining equipment; place the patient in a comfortable position, with the side rails up and the bed in the lowest position.	
——	——	——	25. Remove PPE, if used. Perform hand hygiene.	
——	——	——	26. Check all wound dressings every shift. More frequent checks may be needed if the wound is more complex or dressings become saturated quickly.	

Skill Checklists for Fundamentals of Nursing:
The Art and Science of Person-Centered Nursing Care, 8th edition

Name _____   Date _____

Unit _____   Position _____

Instructor/Evaluator: _____   Position _____

Excellent	Satisfactory	Needs Practice	SKILL 31-3 **Performing Irrigation of a Wound**	Comments
			Goal: The wound is cleaned without contamination or trauma and without causing the patient to experience pain or discomfort.	
___	___	___	1. Review the medical orders for wound care or the nursing plan of care related to wound care. Gather the necessary supplies.	
___	___	___	2. Perform hand hygiene and put on PPE, if indicated.	
___	___	___	3. Identify the patient.	
___	___	___	4. Assemble the equipment on the overbed table within reach.	
___	___	___	5. Close the curtains around the bed and close the door to the room if possible. Explain what you are going to do and why you are going to do it to the patient.	
			6. Assess the patient for the possible need for nonpharmacologic pain-reducing interventions or analgesic medication before wound care and/or dressing change. Administer the appropriate prescribed analgesic. Allow enough time for the analgesic to achieve its effectiveness before beginning the procedure.	
___	___	___	7. Place a waste receptacle or bag at a convenient location for use during the procedure.	
___	___	___	8. Adjust the bed to a comfortable working height, usually elbow height of the caregiver.	
___	___	___	9. Assist the patient to a comfortable position that provides easy access to the wound area. Position the patient so that the irrigation solution will flow from the clean end of the wound toward the dirtier end. Use the bath blanket to cover any exposed area other than the wound. Place a waterproof pad under the wound site.	
___	___	___	10. Put on a gown, mask, and eye protection.	
___	___	___	11. Put on clean gloves. Carefully and gently remove the soiled dressings. If there is resistance, use a silicone-based adhesive remover to help remove the tape. If any part of the dressing sticks to the underlying skin, use small amounts of sterile saline to help loosen and remove it.	
___	___	___	12. After removing the dressing, note the presence, amount, type, color, and odor of any drainage on the dressings. Place soiled dressings in the appropriate waste receptacle.	

Performing Irrigation of a Wound (Continued)

Excellent	Satisfactory	Needs Practice		Comments
——	——	——	13. Assess the wound for appearance, stage, presence of eschar, granulation tissue, epithelialization, undermining, tunneling, necrosis, sinus tract, and drainage. Assess the appearance of the surrounding tissue. Measure the wound.	
——	——	——	14. Remove your gloves and put them in the receptacle.	
——	——	——	15. Set up a sterile field, if indicated, and wound cleaning supplies. Pour warmed sterile irrigating solution into the sterile container. Put on the sterile gloves. Alternately, clean gloves (clean technique) may be used when irrigating a chronic wound or pressure ulcer.	
——	——	——	16. Position the sterile basin below the wound to collect the irrigation fluid.	
——	——	——	17. Fill the irrigation syringe with solution. *Using your nondominant hand, gently apply pressure to the basin against the skin below the wound to form a seal with the skin.*	
——	——	——	18. *Gently direct a stream of solution into the wound. Keep the tip of the syringe at least 1 inch above the upper tip of the wound. When using a catheter tip, insert it gently into the wound until it meets resistance. Gently flush all wound areas.*	
——	——	——	19. Watch for the solution to flow smoothly and evenly. When the solution from the wound flows out clear, discontinue irrigation.	
——	——	——	20. Dry the surrounding skin with gauze dressings.	
——	——	——	21. Apply a skin protectant to the surrounding skin.	
——	——	——	22. Apply a new dressing to the wound.	
——	——	——	23. Remove and discard gloves. Apply tape, Montgomery straps, or roller gauze to secure the dressings. Alternately, many commercial wound products are self-adhesive and do not require additional tape.	
——	——	——	24. After securing the dressing, label it with date and time. Remove all remaining equipment; place the patient in a comfortable position, with side rails up and bed in the lowest position.	
——	——	——	25. Remove remaining PPE. Perform hand hygiene.	
——	——	——	26. Check all wound dressings every shift. More frequent checks may be needed if the wound is more complex or dressings become saturated quickly.	

Skill Checklists for Fundamentals of Nursing:
The Art and Science of Person-Centered Nursing Care, 8th edition

Name _____   Date _____

Unit _____   Position _____

Instructor/Evaluator: _____   Position _____

SKILL 31-4

Caring for a Jackson-Pratt Drain

Excellent	Satisfactory	Needs Practice	**Goal:** The drain is patent and intact.	Comments
⎯	⎯	⎯	1. Review the medical orders for wound care or the nursing plan of care related to wound/drain care. Gather necessary supplies.	
⎯	⎯	⎯	2. Perform hand hygiene and put on PPE, if indicated.	
⎯	⎯	⎯	3. Identify the patient.	
⎯	⎯	⎯	4. Assemble equipment on the overbed table within reach.	
⎯	⎯	⎯	5. Close the curtains around the bed and close the door to the room, if possible. Explain what you are going to do and why you are going to do it to the patient.	
⎯	⎯	⎯	6. Assess the patient for possible need for nonpharmacologic pain-reducing interventions or analgesic medication before wound care dressing change. Administer the appropriate prescribed analgesic. Allow enough time for the analgesic to achieve its effectiveness before beginning the procedure.	
⎯	⎯	⎯	7. Place a waste receptacle at a convenient location for use during the procedure.	
⎯	⎯	⎯	8. Adjust the bed to a comfortable working height, usually elbow height of the caregiver.	
⎯	⎯	⎯	9. Assist the patient to a comfortable position that provides easy access to the drain and/or wound area. Use a bath blanket to cover any exposed area other than the wound. Place a waterproof pad under the wound site.	
⎯	⎯	⎯	10. Put on clean gloves; put on a mask or face shield, as indicated.	
⎯	⎯	⎯	11. Place the graduated collection container under the drain outlet. Without contaminating the outlet valve, pull off the cap. The chamber will expand completely as it draws in air. *Empty the chamber's contents completely into the container. Use the gauze pad to clean the outlet. Fully compress the chamber with one hand and replace the cap with your other hand.*	
⎯	⎯	⎯	12. Check the patency of the equipment. *Make sure the tubing is free from twists and kinks.*	

SKILL 31-4

Caring for a Jackson-Pratt Drain *(Continued)*

Excellent	Satisfactory	Needs Practice		Comments
——	——	——	13. Secure the Jackson-Pratt drain to the patient's gown below the wound with a safety pin, ***making sure that there is no tension on the tubing.***	
——	——	——	14. Carefully measure and record the character, color, and amount of the drainage. Discard the drainage according to facility policy. Remove gloves.	
——	——	——	15. Put on clean gloves. If the drain site has a dressing, redress the site. Include cleaning of the sutures with the gauze pad moistened with normal saline. Dry sutures with gauze before applying the new dressing.	
——	——	——	16. If the drain site is open to air, observe the sutures that secure the drain to the skin. Look for signs of pulling, tearing, swelling, or infection of the surrounding skin. Gently clean the sutures with the gauze pad moistened with normal saline. Dry with a new gauze pad. Apply skin protectant to the surrounding skin, if needed.	
——	——	——	17. Remove and discard gloves. Remove all remaining equipment; place the patient in a comfortable position, with the side rails up and the bed in the lowest position.	
——	——	——	18. Remove additional PPE, if used. Perform hand hygiene.	
——	——	——	19. Check drain status at least every 4 hours. Check all wound dressings every shift. Perform more frequent checks if the wound is more complex or dressings become saturated quickly.	

Skill Checklists for Fundamentals of Nursing:
The Art and Science of Person-Centered Nursing Care, 8th edition

Name _____   Date _____

Unit _____   Position _____

Instructor/Evaluator: _____   Position _____

Excellent	Satisfactory	Needs Practice	SKILL 31-5 **Caring for a Hemovac Drain**	
			Goal: The drain is patent and intact.	**Comments**
——	——	——	1. Review the medical orders for wound care or the nursing plan of care related to wound/drain care. Gather necessary supplies.	
——	——	——	2. Perform hand hygiene and put on PPE, if indicated.	
——	——	——	3. Identify the patient.	
——	——	——	4. Assemble equipment on the overbed table within reach.	
——	——	——	5. Close curtains around the bed and close the door to the room, if possible. Explain what you are going to do and why you are going to do it to the patient.	
——	——	——	6. Assess the patient for the possible need for nonpharmacologic pain-reducing interventions or analgesic medication before wound care dressing change. Administer the appropriate prescribed analgesic. Allow enough time for the analgesic to achieve its effectiveness before beginning the procedure.	
——	——	——	7. Place a waste receptacle at a convenient location for use during the procedure.	
——	——	——	8. Adjust the bed to a comfortable working height, usually elbow height of the caregiver.	
——	——	——	9. Assist the patient to a comfortable position that provides easy access to the drain and/or wound area. Use a bath blanket to cover any exposed area other than the wound. Place a waterproof pad under the wound site.	
——	——	——	10. Put on clean gloves; put on a mask or face shield, as indicated.	
——	——	——	11. Place the graduated collection container under the drain outlet. *Without contaminating the outlet, pull off the cap.* The chamber will expand completely as it draws in air. *Empty the chamber's contents completely into the container. Use the gauze pad to clean the outlet. Fully compress the chamber by pushing the top and bottom together with your hands. Keep the device tightly compressed while you apply the cap.*	
——	——	——	12. Check the patency of the equipment. *Make sure that the tubing is free from twists and kinks.*	

SKILL 31-5

Caring for a Hemovac Drain *(Continued)*

Excellent	Satisfactory	Needs Practice		Comments
——	——	——	13. Secure the Hemovac drain to the patient's gown below the wound with a safety pin, ***making sure that there is no tension on the tubing.***	
——	——	——	14. Carefully measure and record the character, color, and amount of the drainage. Discard the drainage according to facility policy.	
——	——	——	15. Put on clean gloves. If the drain site has a dressing, redress the site. Include cleaning of the sutures with the gauze pad moistened with normal saline. Dry sutures with gauze before applying new dressing.	
——	——	——	16. If the drain site is open to air, observe the sutures that secure the drain to the skin. Look for signs of pulling, tearing, swelling, or infection of the surrounding skin. Gently clean the sutures with the gauze pad moistened with normal saline. Dry with a new gauze pad. Apply skin protectant to the surrounding skin, if needed.	
——	——	——	17. Remove and discard gloves. Remove all remaining equipment; place the patient in a comfortable position, with the side rails up and the bed in the lowest position.	
——	——	——	18. Remove additional PPE, if used. Perform hand hygiene.	
——	——	——	19. Check drain status at least every 4 hours. Check all wound dressings every shift. More frequent checks may be needed if the wound is more complex or dressings become saturated quickly.	

Skill Checklists for Fundamentals of Nursing:
The Art and Science of Person-Centered Nursing Care, 8th edition

Name _____   Date _____

Unit _____   Position _____

Instructor/Evaluator: _____   Position _____

SKILL 31-6

Collecting a Wound Culture

Excellent	Satisfactory	Needs Practice		Comments
			Goal: The culture is obtained without evidence of contamination, without exposing the patient to additional pathogens, and without causing discomfort for the patient.	
⎯⎯	⎯⎯	⎯⎯	1. Review the medical orders for obtaining a wound culture. Gather necessary supplies.	
⎯⎯	⎯⎯	⎯⎯	2. Perform hand hygiene and put on PPE, if indicated.	
⎯⎯	⎯⎯	⎯⎯	3. Identify the patient.	
⎯⎯	⎯⎯	⎯⎯	4. Assemble equipment on the overbed table within reach.	
⎯⎯	⎯⎯	⎯⎯	5. Close curtains around the bed and close the door to the room if possible. Explain what you are going to do and why you are going to do it to the patient.	
⎯⎯	⎯⎯	⎯⎯	6. Assess the patient for the possible need for nonpharmacologic pain-reducing interventions or analgesic medication before obtaining the wound culture. Administer the appropriate prescribed analgesic. Allow enough time for the analgesic to achieve its effectiveness before beginning the procedure.	
⎯⎯	⎯⎯	⎯⎯	7. Place an appropriate waste receptacle within easy reach for use during the procedure.	
⎯⎯	⎯⎯	⎯⎯	8. Adjust the bed to a comfortable working height, usually elbow height of the caregiver.	
⎯⎯	⎯⎯	⎯⎯	9. Assist the patient to a comfortable position that provides easy access to the wound. If necessary, drape the patient with the bath blanket to expose only the wound area. Place a waterproof pad under the wound site. Check the culture label against the patient's identification bracelet.	
⎯⎯	⎯⎯	⎯⎯	10. If there is a dressing in place on the wound, put on clean gloves. Carefully and gently remove the soiled dressings. If there is resistance, use a silicone-based adhesive remover to help remove the tape. If any part of the dressing sticks to the underlying skin, use small amounts of sterile saline to help loosen and remove it.	
⎯⎯	⎯⎯	⎯⎯	11. After removing the dressing, note the presence, amount, type, color, and odor of any drainage on the dressings. Place soiled dressings in the appropriate waste receptacle.	
⎯⎯	⎯⎯	⎯⎯	12. Assess the wound for appearance, stage, presence of eschar, granulation tissue, epithelialization, undermining, tunneling, necrosis, sinus tract, and drainage. Assess the appearance of the surrounding tissue. Measure the wound.	

SKILL 31-6

Collecting a Wound Culture *(Continued)*

Excellent	Satisfactory	Needs Practice		Comments
___	___	___	13. Remove your gloves and put them in the receptacle.	
___	___	___	14. Set up a sterile field, if indicated, and wound cleaning supplies. Put on the sterile gloves. Alternately, clean gloves (clean technique) may be used when cleaning a chronic wound.	
___	___	___	15. Clean the wound. Alternately, irrigate the wound, as ordered or required.	
___	___	___	16. Dry the surrounding skin with gauze dressings. Put on clean gloves.	
___	___	___	17. Twist the cap to loosen the swab on the Culturette tube, or open the separate swab and remove the cap from the culture tube. *Keep the swab and inside of the culture tube sterile.*	
___	___	___	18. If contact with the wound is necessary to separate wound margins to permit insertion of the swab deep into the wound, put a sterile glove on one hand to manipulate the wound margins. Clean gloves may be appropriate for contact with pressure ulcers and chronic wounds.	
___	___	___	19. *Carefully insert the swab into the wound. Press and rotate the swab several times over the wound surfaces. Avoid touching the swab to intact skin at the wound edges. Use another swab if collecting a specimen from another site.*	
___	___	___	20. Place the swab back in the culture tube. *Do not touch the outside of the tube with the swab.* Secure the cap. Some swab containers have an ampule of medium at the bottom of the tube. It might be necessary to crush this ampule to activate. Follow the manufacturer's instructions for use.	
___	___	___	21. Remove gloves and discard them accordingly.	
___	___	___	22. Put on gloves. Place a dressing on the wound, as appropriate, based on medical orders and/or the nursing plan of care.	
___	___	___	23. After securing the dressing, label the dressing with the date and time. Remove all remaining equipment; place the patient in a comfortable position, with the side rails up and the bed in the lowest position.	
___	___	___	24. Label the specimen according to your institution's guidelines and send it to the laboratory in a biohazard bag.	
___	___	___	25. Remove PPE, if used. Perform hand hygiene.	

Skill Checklists for Fundamentals of Nursing:
The Art and Science of Person-Centered Nursing Care, 8th edition

Name _____ Date _____

Unit _____ Position _____

Instructor/Evaluator: _____ Position _____

SKILL 31-7
Applying Negative-Pressure Wound Therapy

Goal: The therapy is accomplished without contaminating the wound area, without causing trauma to the wound, and without causing the patient to experience pain or discomfort.

Excellent	Satisfactory	Needs Practice		Comments
___	___	___	1. Review the medical order for the application of NPWT therapy, including the ordered pressure setting for the device. Gather necessary supplies.	
___	___	___	2. Perform hand hygiene and put on PPE, if indicated.	
___	___	___	3. Identify the patient.	
___	___	___	4. Assemble equipment on the overbed table within reach.	
___	___	___	5. Close curtains around the bed and close the door to the room, if possible. Explain what you are going to do and why you are going to do it to the patient.	
___	___	___	6. Assess the patient for the possible need for nonpharmacologic pain-reducing interventions or analgesic medication before wound care dressing change. Administer the appropriate prescribed analgesic. Allow enough time for the analgesic to achieve its effectiveness before beginning the procedure.	
___	___	___	7. Adjust the bed to a comfortable working height, usually elbow height of the caregiver.	
___	___	___	8. Assist the patient to a comfortable position that provides easy access to the wound area. Position the patient so that the irrigation solution will flow from the clean end of the wound toward the dirty end. Expose the area and drape the patient with a bath blanket if needed. Put a waterproof pad under the wound area.	
___	___	___	9. Have the disposal bag or waste receptacle within easy reach for use during the procedure.	
___	___	___	10. Using sterile technique, prepare a sterile field and add all the sterile supplies needed for the procedure to the field. Pour warmed, sterile irrigating solution into the sterile container.	
___	___	___	11. Put on a gown, mask, and eye protection.	
___	___	___	12. Put on clean gloves. Carefully and gently remove the dressing. If there is resistance, use a silicone-based adhesive remover to help remove the dressing. *Note the number of pieces of foam removed from the wound. Compare with the documented number from the previous dressing change.*	

Excellent	Satisfactory	Needs Practice		Comments

SKILL 31-7

Applying Negative-Pressure Wound Therapy *(Continued)*

Excellent	Satisfactory	Needs Practice		
____	____	____	13. Discard the dressings in the receptacle. Remove your gloves and put them in the receptacle.	
____	____	____	14. Put on sterile gloves. Using sterile technique, irrigate the wound.	
____	____	____	15. Clean the area around the wound with normal saline. Dry the surrounding skin with a sterile gauze sponge.	
____	____	____	16. Assess the wound for appearance, stage, the presence of eschar, granulation tissue, epithelialization, undermining, tunneling, necrosis, sinus tract, and drainage. Assess the appearance of the surrounding tissue. Measure the wound.	
____	____	____	17. *Wipe intact skin around the wound with a skin-protectant wipe and allow it to dry well.*	
____	____	____	18. *Using sterile scissors, cut the foam to the shape and measurement of the wound. Do not cut foam over the wound.* More than one piece of foam may be necessary if the first piece is cut too small. Carefully place the foam in the wound. *Ensure foam-to-foam contact if more than one piece is required. Note the number of pieces of foam placed in the wound.*	
____	____	____	19. Trim and place the V.A.C. Drape to cover the foam dressing and an additional 3- to 5-cm border of intact peri-wound tissue. The V.A.C. Drape may be cut into multiple pieces for easier handling.	
____	____	____	20. Choose an appropriate site to apply the T.R.A.C. Pad.	
____	____	____	21. Pinch the drape and cut a 2-cm hole through it. Apply the T.R.A.C. Pad. Remove V.A.C. Canister from the package and insert into the V.A.C. Therapy Unit until it locks into place. Connect the T.R.A.C. Pad tubing to canister tubing and check that the clamps on each tube are open. Turn on the power to the V.A.C. Therapy Unit and select the prescribed therapy setting.	
____	____	____	22. *Assess the dressing to ensure seal integrity. The dressing should be collapsed, shrinking to the foam and skin.*	
____	____	____	23. Remove and discard gloves.	
____	____	____	24. Label the dressing with the date and time. Remove all remaining equipment; place the patient in a comfortable position, with the side rails up and the bed in the lowest position.	
____	____	____	25. Remove PPE, if used. Perform hand hygiene.	
____	____	____	26. Check all wound dressings every shift. More frequent checks may be needed if the wound is more complex or dressings become saturated quickly.	

Skill Checklists for Fundamentals of Nursing:
The Art and Science of Person-Centered Nursing Care, 8th edition

Name _____   Date _____

Unit _____   Position _____

Instructor/Evaluator: _____   Position _____

Excellent	Satisfactory	Needs Practice	SKILL 31-8 **Applying an External Heating Pad**	Comments
			Goal: Desired outcome depends on the patient's nursing diagnosis.	
___	___	___	1. Review the medical order for the application of heat therapy, including frequency, type of therapy, body area to be treated, and length of time for the application. Gather necessary supplies.	
___	___	___	2. Perform hand hygiene and put on PPE, if indicated.	
___	___	___	3. Identify the patient.	
___	___	___	4. Assemble equipment on the overbed table within reach.	
___	___	___	5. Close the curtains around the bed and the close door to the room, if possible. Explain what you are going to do and why you are going to do it to the patient.	
___	___	___	6. Adjust the bed to a comfortable working height, usually elbow height of the caregiver.	
___	___	___	7. Assist the patient to a comfortable position that provides easy access to the area where the heat will be applied; use a bath blanket to cover any other exposed area.	
___	___	___	8. Assess the condition of the skin where the heat is to be applied.	
___	___	___	9. Check that the water in the electronic unit is at the appropriate level. Fill the unit two-thirds full or to the fill mark, with distilled water, if necessary. Check the temperature setting on the unit to ensure that it is within the safe range.	
___	___	___	10. Attach the pad tubing to the electronic unit tubing.	
___	___	___	11. Plug in the unit and warm the pad before use. Apply the heating pad to the prescribed area. Secure with gauze bandage or tape.	
___	___	___	12. *Assess the condition of the skin and the patient's response to the heat at frequent intervals, according to facility policy. Do not exceed the prescribed length of time for the application of heat.*	
___	___	___	13. Remove gloves and discard. Remove all remaining equipment; place the patient in a comfortable position, with the side rails up and the bed in the lowest position.	
___	___	___	14. Remove additional PPE, if used. Perform hand hygiene.	

Applying an External Heating Pad *(Continued)*

Excellent	Satisfactory	Needs Practice		Comments
——	——	——	15. *Monitor the time the heating pad is in place to prevent burns and skin/tissue damage. Monitor the condition of the patient's skin and the patient's response at frequent intervals.*	
——	——	——	16. Remove the pad after the prescribed amount of time (up to 30 minutes). Reassess the patient and area of application, noting the effect and presence of adverse effects.	

Skill Checklists for Fundamentals of Nursing:
The Art and Science of Person-Centered Nursing Care, 8th edition

Name _____ Date _____

Unit _____ Position _____

Instructor/Evaluator: _____ Position _____

Excellent	Satisfactory	Needs Practice	SKILL 32-1 **Applying and Removing Graduated Compression Stockings**	
			Goal: The stockings will be applied and removed with minimal discomfort to the patient.	**Comments**
___	___	___	1. Review the medical record and medical orders to determine the need for graduated compression stockings.	
___	___	___	2. Perform hand hygiene. Put on PPE, as indicated.	
___	___	___	3. Identify the patient. Explain what you are going to do and the rationale for use of elastic stockings.	
___	___	___	4. Close the curtains around the bed and close the door to the room, if possible.	
___	___	___	5. Adjust the bed to a comfortable working height, usually elbow height of the caregiver.	
___	___	___	6. Assist the patient to the supine position. If the patient has been sitting or walking, have the patient lie down with legs and feet well elevated for at least 15 minutes before applying stockings.	
___	___	___	7. Expose legs one at a time. Wash and dry legs, if necessary. Powder the leg lightly unless the patient has a respiratory problem, dry skin, or sensitivity to the powder. If the skin is dry, a lotion may be used. Powders and lotions are not recommended by some manufacturers; check the package material for manufacturer specifications.	
___	___	___	8. Stand at the foot of the bed. Place a hand inside the stocking and grasp the heel area securely. Turn the stocking inside-out to the heel area, leaving the foot inside the stocking leg.	
___	___	___	9. With the heel pocket down, ease the stocking foot over the foot and heel. Check that the patient's heel is centered in the heel pocket of the stocking.	
___	___	___	10. Using your fingers and thumbs, carefully grasp the edge of the stocking and pull it up smoothly over the ankle and calf, toward the knee. Make sure it is distributed evenly.	
___	___	___	11. Pull forward slightly on the toe section. If the stocking has a toe window, make sure it is properly positioned. Adjust if necessary to ensure that the material is smooth.	

SKILL 32-1

Applying and Removing Graduated Compression Stockings *(Continued)*

Excellent	Satisfactory	Needs Practice		Comments
____	____	____	12. If the stockings are knee-length, make sure each stocking top is 1 to 2 inches below the patella. Make sure the stocking does not roll down.	
____	____	____	13. If applying thigh-length stocking, continue the application. Flex the patient's leg. Stretch the stocking over the knee.	
____	____	____	14. Pull the stocking over the thigh until the top is 1 to 3 inches below the gluteal fold. Adjust the stocking, as necessary, to distribute the fabric evenly. Make sure the stocking does not roll down.	
____	____	____	15. Remove equipment and return the patient to a position of comfort. Remove gloves. Raise the side rail and lower the bed. Place the call bell and other essential items within reach.	
____	____	____	16. Remove any other PPE, if used. Perform hand hygiene.	
			Removing Stockings	
____	____	____	17. To remove a stocking, grasp the top of the stocking with your thumb and fingers and smoothly pull the stocking off inside out to heel. Support the foot and ease the stocking over it.	

Skill Checklists for Fundamentals of Nursing:
The Art and Science of Person-Centered Nursing Care, 8th edition

Name _____ Date _____

Unit _____ Position _____

Instructor/Evaluator: _____ Position _____

Excellent	Satisfactory	Needs Practice	SKILL 32-2 **Assisting a Patient With Turning in Bed**	
			Goal: The activity takes place without injury to patient or nurse.	**Comments**
___	___	___	1. Review the medical orders and nursing plan of care for patient activity. Identify any movement limitations and the ability of the patient to assist with turning. ***Consult patient handling algorithm, if available, to plan appropriate approach to moving the patient.***	
___	___	___	2. Gather any positioning aids or supports, if necessary.	
___	___	___	3. Perform hand hygiene. Put on PPE, as indicated.	
___	___	___	4. Identify the patient. Explain the procedure to the patient.	
___	___	___	5. Close the curtains around the bed and close the door to the room, if possible. Position at least one nurse on either side of the bed. Place pillows, wedges, or any other support to be used for positioning within easy reach. Place the bed at an appropriate and comfortable working height, usually elbow height of the caregiver. Lower both side rails.	
___	___	___	6. If not already in place, position a friction-reducing sheet under the patient.	
___	___	___	7. Using the friction-reducing sheet, move the patient to the edge of the bed, opposite the side to which the patient will be turned. Raise the side rails.	
___	___	___	8. If the patient is able, have the patient grasp the side rail on the side of the bed toward which the patient is turning. Alternately, place the patient's arms across his or her chest and cross his or her far leg over the leg toward which they are turning.	
___	___	___	9. If available, activate the bed turn mechanism to inflate the side of the bed behind the patient's back.	

SKILL 32-2

Assisting a Patient With Turning in Bed *(Continued)*

Excellent	Satisfactory	Needs Practice		Comments
——	——	——	10. The nurse on the side of the bed toward which the patient is turning should stand opposite the patient's center with feet spread about shoulder width and with one foot ahead of the other. Tighten your gluteal and abdominal muscles and flex your knees. Use your leg muscles to do the pulling. The other nurse should position hands on the patient's shoulder and hip, assisting to roll the patient to the side. Instruct the patient to pull on the bed rail at the same time. Use the friction-reducing sheet to gently pull the patient over on his or her side.	
——	——	——	11. Use a pillow or other support behind the patient's back. Pull the shoulder blade forward and out from under the patient.	
——	——	——	12. Make the patient comfortable and position in proper alignment, using pillows or other supports under the leg and arm, as needed. Readjust the pillow under the patient's head. Elevate the head of the bed as needed for comfort.	
——	——	——	13. Place the bed in the lowest position, with the side rails up, as indicated. Make sure the call bell and other necessary items are within easy reach.	
——	——	——	14. Clean transfer aids, per facility policy, if not indicated for single patient use. Remove gloves and other PPE, if used. Perform hand hygiene.	

Skill Checklists for Fundamentals of Nursing:
The Art and Science of Person-Centered Nursing Care, 8th edition

Name _____ Date _____

Unit _____ Position _____

Instructor/Evaluator: _____ Position _____

			SKILL 32-3	
Excellent	**Satisfactory**	**Needs Practice**	**Moving a Patient Up in Bed With the Assistance of Another Caregiver** **Goal:** The patient remains free from injury and maintains proper body alignment.	**Comments**
___ ___ ___			1. Review the medical record and nursing plan of care for conditions that may influence the patient's ability to move or to be positioned. Assess for tubes, IV lines, incisions, or equipment that may alter the positioning procedure. Identify any movement limitations. ***Consult patient handling algorithm, if available, to plan appropriate approach to moving the patient.***	
___ ___ ___			2. Perform hand hygiene and put on PPE, if indicated.	
___ ___ ___			3. Identify the patient. Explain the procedure to the patient.	
___ ___ ___			4. Close the curtains around the bed and close the door to the room, if possible. Place the bed at an appropriate and comfortable working height, usually elbow height of the caregiver. Adjust the head of the bed to a flat position or as low as the patient can tolerate. Place the bed in slight Trendelenburg position, if the patient is able to tolerate it.	
___ ___ ___			5. Remove all pillows from under the patient. Leave one at the head of the bed, leaning upright against the headboard.	
___ ___ ___			6. Position at least one nurse on either side of the bed, and lower both side rails.	
___ ___ ___			7. If a friction-reducing sheet (or device) is not in place under the patient, place one under the patient's midsection.	
___ ___ ___			8. Ask the patient (if able) to bend the legs and put feet flat on the bed to assist with the movement.	
___ ___ ___			9. Have the patient fold the arms across the chest. Have the patient (if able) lift the head, with the chin on the chest.	
___ ___ ___			10. One nurse should be positioned on each side of the bed, at the patient's midsection, with feet spread shoulder width apart and one foot slightly in front of the other.	
___ ___ ___			11. If available on the bed, engage the mechanism to make the bed surface firmer for repositioning.	
___ ___ ___			12. Grasp the friction-reducing sheet securely, close to the patient's body.	
___ ___ ___			13. Flex your knees and hips. Tighten your abdominal and gluteal muscles, and keep your back straight.	

SKILL 32-3

Moving a Patient Up in Bed With the Assistance of Another Caregiver *(Continued)*

Excellent	Satisfactory	Needs Practice		Comments
___	___	___	14. If possible, the patient can assist with the move by pushing with the legs. Shift your weight back and forth from your back leg to your front leg and count to three. On the count of three, move the patient up in bed. Repeat the process, if necessary, to get the patient to the right position.	
___	___	___	15. Assist the patient to a comfortable position and readjust the pillows and supports, as needed. Take the bed out of Trendelenburg position and return the bed surface to the normal setting, if necessary. Raise the side rails. Place the bed in the lowest position. Make sure the call bell and other necessary items are within easy reach.	
___	___	___	16. Clean transfer aids per facility policy, if not indicated for single-patient use. Remove gloves or other PPE, if used. Perform hand hygiene.	

Skill Checklists for Fundamentals of Nursing:
The Art and Science of Person-Centered Nursing Care, 8th edition

Name _____   Date _____

Unit _____   Position _____

Instructor/Evaluator: _____   Position _____

	SKILL 32-4	
	Transferring a Patient From the Bed to a Stretcher	

Excellent	Satisfactory	Needs Practice	**Goal:** The patient is transferred without injury to patient or nurse.	**Comments**
____	____	____	1. Review the medical record and nursing plan of care for conditions that may influence the patient's ability to move or to be positioned. Assess for tubes, IV lines, incisions, or equipment that may alter the positioning procedure. Identify any movement limitations. *Consult patient handling algorithm, if available, to plan appropriate approach to moving the patient.*	
____	____	____	2. Perform hand hygiene and put on PPE, if indicated.	
____	____	____	3. Identify the patient. Explain the procedure to the patient.	
____	____	____	4. Close curtains around the bed and close the door to the room, if possible. Adjust the head of the bed to a flat position or as low as the patient can tolerate. Raise the bed to a height that is even with the transport stretcher. Lower the side rails, if in place.	
____	____	____	5. Place the bath blanket over the patient and remove the top covers from underneath.	
____	____	____	6. If a friction-reducing transfer sheet is not in place under the patient, place one under the patient's midsection. Have the patient fold the arms against the chest and move the chin to the chest. Use the friction-reducing sheet to move the patient to the side of the bed where the stretcher will be placed. Alternately, place a lateral-assist device under the patient. Follow the manufacturer's directions for use.	
____	____	____	7. Position the stretcher next to (and parallel) to the bed. *Lock the wheels on the stretcher and the bed.*	
____	____	____	8. Two nurses should stand on the stretcher side of the bed. A third nurse should stand on the side of the bed without the stretcher.	
____	____	____	9. Use the friction-reducing sheet to roll the patient away from the stretcher. Place the transfer board across the space between the stretcher and the bed, partially under the patient. Roll the patient onto his or her back, so that the patient is partially on the transfer board.	

SKILL 32-4

Transferring a Patient From the
Bed to a Stretcher *(Continued)*

Excellent	Satisfactory	Needs Practice		Comments
——	——	——	10. The nurse on the side of the bed without the stretcher should grasp the friction-reducing sheet at the head and chest areas of the patient. The nurse on the stretcher side of the bed should grasp the friction-reducing sheet at the head and chest, and the other nurse on that side should grasp the friction-reducing sheet at the chest and leg areas of the patient.	
——	——	——	11. *At a signal given by one of the nurses, have the nurses standing on the stretcher side of the bed pull the friction-reducing sheet. At the same time, the nurse (or nurses) on the other side push, transferring the patient's weight toward the transfer board, and pushing the patient from the bed to the stretcher.*	
——	——	——	12. Once the patient is transferred to the stretcher, remove the transfer board, and secure the patient until the side rails are raised. Raise the side rails. To ensure the patient's comfort, cover the patient with a blanket and remove the bath blanket from underneath. Leave the friction-reducing sheet in place for the return transfer. Make sure the call bell and other necessary items are within easy reach.	
——	——	——	13. Clean the transfer aids per facility policy, if not indicated for single-patient use. Remove gloves and any other PPE, if used. Perform hand hygiene.	

Skill Checklists for Fundamentals of Nursing:
The Art and Science of Person-Centered Nursing Care, 8th edition

Name _____ Date _____

Unit _____ Position _____

Instructor/Evaluator: _____ Position _____

SKILL 32-5

Transferring a Patient From the Bed to a Chair

Goal: The transfer is accomplished without injury to patient or nurse and the patient remains free of any complications of immobility.

Excellent	Satisfactory	Needs Practice		Comments
⎯	⎯	⎯	1. Review the medical record and nursing plan of care for conditions that may influence the patient's ability to move or to be positioned. Assess for tubes, IV lines, incisions, or equipment that may alter the positioning procedure. Identify any movement limitations. *Consult patient-handling algorithm, if available, to plan appropriate approach to moving the patient.*	
⎯	⎯	⎯	2. Perform hand hygiene and put on PPE, as indicated.	
⎯	⎯	⎯	3. Identify the patient. Explain the procedure to the patient.	
⎯	⎯	⎯	4. If needed, move equipment to make room for the chair. Close the curtains around the bed and close the door to the room, if possible.	
⎯	⎯	⎯	5. Place the bed in the lowest position. Raise the head of the bed to a sitting position, or as high as the patient can tolerate.	
⎯	⎯	⎯	6. *Make sure the bed brakes are locked. Put the chair next to the bed. If available, lock the brakes of the chair. If the chair does not have brakes, brace the chair against a secure object.*	
⎯	⎯	⎯	7. Encourage the patient to make use of a stand-assist aid, either freestanding or attached to the side of the bed, if available, to move to the side of the bed and to a side-lying position, facing the side of the bed on which the patient will sit.	
⎯	⎯	⎯	8. Lower the side rail, if necessary, and stand near the patient's hips. Stand with your legs shoulder width apart with one foot near the head of the bed, slightly in front of the other foot.	
⎯	⎯	⎯	9. Encourage the patient to make use of the stand-assist device. Assist the patient to sit up on the side of the bed; ask the patient to swing the legs over the side of the bed. At the same time, pivot on your back leg to lift the patient's trunk and shoulders. Keep your back straight; avoid twisting.	

Transferring a Patient From the Bed to a Chair *(Continued)*

Excellent	Satisfactory	Needs Practice		Comments
——	——	——	10. *Stand in front of the patient, and assess for any balance problems or complaints of dizziness. Allow the patient's legs to dangle a few minutes before continuing.*	
——	——	——	11. Assist the patient to put on a robe, as necessary, and non-skid footwear.	
——	——	——	12. Wrap the gait belt around the patient's waist, based on assessed need and facility policy.	
——	——	——	13. Stand facing the patient. Spread your feet about shoulder width apart and flex your hips and knees.	
——	——	——	14. Ask the patient to slide the buttocks to the edge of the bed until the feet touch the floor. Position yourself as close as possible to the patient, with your foot positioned on the outside of the patient's foot. If a second staff person is assisting, have that staff person assume a similar position. Grasp the gait belt.	
——	——	——	15. Encourage the patient to make use of the stand-assist device. If necessary, have the second staff person grasp the gait belt on the opposite side. Rock back and forth while counting to three. *On the count of three, using the gait belt and your legs (not your back), assist the patient to a standing position.* If indicated, brace your front knee against the patient's weak extremity as the patient stands. Assess the patient's balance and leg strength. If the patient is weak or unsteady, return the patient to bed.	
——	——	——	16. Pivot on your back foot and assist the patient to turn until the patient feels the chair against his or her legs.	
——	——	——	17. Ask the patient to use his arm to steady himself on the arm of the chair while slowly lowering to a sitting position. Continue to brace the patient's knees with your knees and hold the gait belt. Flex your hips and knees when helping the patient sit in the chair.	
——	——	——	18. Assess the patient's alignment in the chair. Remove the gait belt, if desired. Depending on patient comfort, it could be left in place to use when returning to bed. Cover with a blanket, if needed. Make sure the call bell and other essential items are within easy reach.	
——	——	——	19. Clean transfer aids per facility policy, if not indicated for single-patient use. Remove gloves and any other PPE, if used. Perform hand hygiene.	

Skill Checklists for Fundamentals of Nursing:
The Art and Science of Person-Centered Nursing Care, 8th edition

Name _____ Date _____

Unit _____ Position _____

Instructor/Evaluator: _____ Position _____

Excellent	Satisfactory	Needs Practice	SKILL 32-6 **Providing Range-of-Motion Exercises**	
			Goal: The patient maintains joint mobility.	**Comments**
——	——	——	1. Review the medical orders and nursing plan of care for patient activity. Identify any movement limitations.	
——	——	——	2. Perform hand hygiene and put on PPE, if indicated.	
——	——	——	3. Identify the patient. Explain the procedure to the patient.	
——	——	——	4. Close the curtains around the bed and close the door to the room, if possible. Place the bed at an appropriate and comfortable working height, usually elbow height of the caregiver. Adjust the head of the bed to a flat position or as low as the patient can tolerate.	
——	——	——	5. Stand on the side of the bed where the joints are to be exercised. Lower the side rail on that side, if in place. Uncover only the limb to be used during the exercise.	
——	——	——	6. Perform the exercises slowly and gently, providing support by holding the areas proximal and distal to the joint. Repeat each exercise two to five times, moving each joint in a smooth and rhythmic manner. *Stop movement if the patient complains of pain or if you meet resistance.*	
——	——	——	7. While performing the exercises, begin at the head and move down one side of the body at a time. *Encourage the patient to do as many of these exercises independently as possible.*	
——	——	——	8. Move the chin down to rest on the chest. Return the head to a normal upright position. Tilt the head as far as possible toward each shoulder.	
——	——	——	9. Move the head from side to side, bringing the chin toward each shoulder.	
——	——	——	10. Start with the arm at the patient's side and lift the arm forward to above the head. Return the arm to the starting position at the side of the body.	
——	——	——	11. With the arm back at the patient's side, move the arm laterally to an upright position above the head, and then return it to the original position. Move the arm across the body as far as possible.	

Excellent	Satisfactory	Needs Practice	SKILL 32-6 **Providing Range-of-Motion Exercises** (Continued)	Comments
——	——	——	12. Raise the arm at the side until the upper arm is in line with the shoulder. Bend the elbow at a 90-degree angle and move the forearm upward and downward, then return the arm to the side.	
——	——	——	13. Bend the elbow and move the lower arm and hand upward toward the shoulder. Return the lower arm and hand to the original position while straightening the elbow.	
——	——	——	14. Rotate the lower arm and hand so that the palm is up. Rotate the lower arm and hand so that the palm of the hand is down.	
——	——	——	15. Move the hand downward toward the inner aspect of the forearm. Return the hand to a neutral position even with the forearm. Then move the dorsal portion of the hand backward as far as possible.	
——	——	——	16. Bend the fingers to make a fist, then straighten them out. Spread the fingers apart and return them back together. Touch the thumb to each finger on the hand.	
——	——	——	17. Extend the leg and lift it upward. Return the leg to the original position beside the other leg.	
——	——	——	18. Lift the leg laterally away from the patient's body. Return the leg back toward the other leg and try to extend it beyond the midline.	
——	——	——	19. Turn the foot and leg toward the opposite leg to rotate it internally. Turn the foot and leg outward, away from the opposite leg, to rotate it externally.	
——	——	——	20. Bend the leg and bring the heel toward the back of the leg. Return the leg to a straight position.	
——	——	——	21. At the ankle, move the foot up and back until the toes are upright. Move the foot, with the toes pointing downward.	
——	——	——	22. Turn the sole of the foot toward the midline. Turn the sole of the foot outward.	
——	——	——	23. Curl the toes downward, then straighten them out. Spread the toes apart and bring them together.	
——	——	——	24. Repeat these exercises on the other side of the body. Encourage the patient to do as many of these exercises independently as possible.	
——	——	——	25. When finished, make sure that the patient is comfortable, with the side rails up and the bed in the lowest position. Place the call bell and other essential items within reach.	
——	——	——	26. Remove gloves and any other PPE, if used. Perform hand hygiene.	

Skill Checklists for Fundamentals of Nursing:
The Art and Science of Person-Centered Nursing Care, 8th edition

Name _____   Date _____

Unit _____   Position _____

Instructor/Evaluator: _____   Position _____

SKILL 34-1
Giving a Back Massage

Goal: The patient reports increased comfort and decreased pain, and is relaxed.

Excellent	Satisfactory	Needs Practice		Comments
___	___	___	1. Perform hand hygiene and put on PPE, if indicated.	
___	___	___	2. Identify the patient.	
___	___	___	3. Offer a back massage to the patient and explain the procedure.	
___	___	___	4. Put on gloves, if indicated.	
___	___	___	5. Close the room door and/or the curtain around the bed.	
___	___	___	6. Assess the patient's pain, using an appropriate assessment tool and measurement scale.	
___	___	___	7. Raise the bed to a comfortable working position, usually elbow height of the caregiver, and lower the side rail.	
___	___	___	8. Assist the patient to a comfortable position, preferably the prone or side-lying position. Remove the covers and move the patient's gown just enough to expose the patient's back from the shoulders to sacral area. Drape the patient, as needed, with the bath blanket.	
___	___	___	9. Warm the lubricant or lotion in the palm of your hand, or place the container in a small basin of warm water. *During massage, observe the patient's skin for reddened or open areas. Pay particular attention to the skin over bony prominences.*	
___	___	___	10. Using light, gliding strokes (*effleurage*), apply lotion to patient's shoulders, back, and sacral area.	
___	___	___	11. Place your hands beside each other at the base of the patient's spine and stroke upward to the shoulders and back downward to the buttocks in slow, continuous strokes. Continue for several minutes.	
___	___	___	12. Massage the patient's shoulder, entire back, areas over the iliac crests, and sacrum with circular stroking motions. *Keep your hands in contact with the patient's skin.* Continue for several minutes, applying additional lotion, as necessary.	
___	___	___	13. Knead the patient's skin by gently alternating grasping and compression motions (*pétrissage*).	

SKILL 34-1

Giving a Back Massage *(Continued)*

Excellent	Satisfactory	Needs Practice		Comments
—	—	—	14. Complete the massage with additional long, stroking movements that eventually become lighter in pressure.	
—	—	—	15. Use the towel to pat the patient dry and to remove excess lotion.	
—	—	—	16. Remove gloves, if worn. Reposition the patient's gown and covers. Raise the side rail and lower the bed. Assist the patient to a position of comfort.	
—	—	—	17. Remove additional PPE, if used. Perform hand hygiene.	
—	—	—	18. Evaluate the patient's response to interventions. Reassess the level of discomfort or pain using original assessment tools. Reassess and alter plan of care, as appropriate.	

Skill Checklists for Fundamentals of Nursing:
The Art and Science of Person-Centered Nursing Care, 8th edition

Name _____   Date _____

Unit _____   Position _____

Instructor/Evaluator: _____   Position _____

SKILL 35-1

Inserting a Nasogastric (NG) Tube

Goal: The tube is passed into the patient's stomach without any complications.

Excellent	Satisfactory	Needs Practice		Comments
___	___	___	1. Verify the medical order for insertion of an NG tube. Gather equipment, including selection of the appropriate NG tube.	
___	___	___	2. Perform hand hygiene and put on PPE, if indicated.	
___	___	___	3. Identify the patient.	
___	___	___	4. Explain the procedure to the patient and provide the rationale as to why the tube is needed. Discuss the associated discomforts that may be experienced and possible interventions that may allay this discomfort. Answer any questions as needed.	
___	___	___	5. Assemble equipment on the overbed table within reach.	
___	___	___	6. Close the patient's bedside curtain or door. Raise the bed to a comfortable working position, usually elbow height of the caregiver. Assist the patient to high Fowler's position or elevate the head of the bed 45 degrees if the patient is unable to maintain an upright position. Drape the chest with a bath towel or disposable pad. Have an emesis basin and tissues handy.	
___	___	___	7. *Measure the distance to insert the tube by placing the tip of the tube at the patient's nostril and extending the tube to the tip of the earlobe and then to the tip of the xiphoid process.* Mark the tube with an indelible marker.	
___	___	___	8. Put on gloves. Lubricate the tip of the tube (at least 2 to 4 inches) with water-soluble lubricant. Apply a topical anesthetic to the nostril and oropharynx, as appropriate.	
___	___	___	9. After selecting the appropriate nostril, ask the patient to slightly flex the head back against the pillow. Gently insert the tube into the nostril while directing the tube upward and backward along the floor of the nose. The patient may gag when the tube reaches the pharynx. Provide tissues for tearing or watering of eyes. Offer comfort and reassurance to the patient.	

Inserting a Nasogastric (NG) Tube *(Continued)*

Excellent	Satisfactory	Needs Practice		Comments

10. When the pharynx is reached, instruct the patient to touch the chin to the chest. Encourage the patient to sip water through a straw or swallow even if no fluids are permitted. Advance the tube in a downward and backward direction when the patient swallows. Stop when the patient breathes. *If gagging and coughing persist, stop advancing the tube and check placement of the tube with tongue blade and flashlight.* If the tube is curled, straighten the tube and attempt to advance again. Keep advancing the tube until pen marking is reached. *Do not use force.* Rotate tube if it meets resistance.

11. *Discontinue the procedure and remove the tube if there are signs of distress, such as gasping, coughing, cyanosis, and inability to speak or hum.*

12. Secure the tube loosely to the nose or cheek until it is determined that the tube is in the patient's stomach:

    a. Attach a syringe to the end of the tube and aspirate a small amount of stomach contents.

    b. Measure the pH of the aspirated fluid using pH paper or a meter. Place a drop of gastric secretions onto pH paper or place a small amount in a plastic cup and dip the pH paper into it. Within 30 seconds, compare the color on the paper with the chart supplied by the manufacturer.

    c. Visualize aspirated contents, checking for color and consistency.

    d. Obtain a radiograph (x-ray) of placement of the tube, based on facility policy (and ordered by physician).

13. Apply skin barrier to the tip and end of the nose and allow to dry. Remove gloves and secure the tube with a commercially prepared device (follow manufacturer's directions) or tape to the patient's nose. To secure with tape:

    a. Cut a 4-inch piece of tape and split the bottom 2 inches or use packaged nose tape for NG tubes.

    b. Place the unsplit end over the bridge of the patient's nose.

    c. Wrap split ends under and around the NG tube. *Be careful not to pull the tube too tightly against the nose.*

14. Put on gloves. Clamp the tube and remove the syringe. Cap the tube or attach it to suction according to the medical orders.

SKILL 35-1
Inserting a Nasogastric (NG) Tube *(Continued)*

Excellent	Satisfactory	Needs Practice		Comments
—	—	—	15. Measure length of the exposed tube. Reinforce the marking on the tube at the nostril with indelible ink. Ask the patient to turn the head to the side opposite the nostril in which the tube is inserted. Secure the tube to the patient's gown by using a rubber band or tape and safety pin. For additional support, tape the tube onto the patient's cheek using a piece of tape. *If a double-lumen tube (e.g., Salem sump) is used, secure the vent above the stomach level.* Attach the vent at shoulder level.	
—	—	—	16. Assist with or provide oral hygiene at 2- to 4-hour intervals. Lubricate the lips generously and clean nares and lubricate as needed. Offer analgesic throat lozenges or anesthetic spray for throat irritation if needed.	
—	—	—	17. Remove equipment and return the patient to a position of comfort. Remove gloves. Raise the side rail and lower the bed.	
—	—	—	18. Remove additional PPE, if used. Perform hand hygiene.	

Skill Checklists for Fundamentals of Nursing:
The Art and Science of Person-Centered Nursing Care, 8th edition

Name _____   Date _____

Unit _____   Position _____

Instructor/Evaluator: _____   Position _____

SKILL 35-2

Administering a Tube Feeding

Goal: The patient receives the tube feeding without complaints of nausea or episodes of vomiting.

Excellent	Satisfactory	Needs Practice		Comments
___	___	___	1. Gather equipment. Check amount, concentration, type, and frequency of tube feeding in the patient's medical record. Check expiration date of formula.	
___	___	___	2. Perform hand hygiene and put on PPE, if indicated.	
___	___	___	3. Identify the patient.	
___	___	___	4. Explain the procedure to the patient and why this intervention is needed. Answer any questions as needed.	
___	___	___	5. Assemble equipment on the overbed table within reach.	
___	___	___	6. Close the patient's bedside curtain or door. Raise the bed to a comfortable working position, usually elbow height of the caregiver. Perform key abdominal assessments.	
___	___	___	7. *Position the patient with the head of the bed elevated at least 30 to 45 degrees or as near normal position for eating as possible.*	
___	___	___	8. Put on gloves. Unpin the tube from the patient's gown. Verify the position of the marking on the tube at the nostril. Measure the length of the exposed tube and compare with the documented length.	
___	___	___	9. Attach a syringe to the end of the tube and aspirate a small amount of stomach contents.	
___	___	___	10. Check the pH.	
___	___	___	11. Visualize aspirated contents, checking for color and consistency.	
___	___	___	12. If it is not possible to aspirate contents, assessments to check placement are inconclusive, the exposed tube length has changed, or there are any other indications that the tube is not in place, check placement by x-ray.	
___	___	___	13. After multiple steps have been taken to ensure that the feeding tube is located in the stomach or small intestine, *aspirate all gastric contents with the syringe and measure to check for gastric residual—the amount of feeding remaining in the stomach.* Return the residual based on facility policy. Proceed with feeding if amount of residual does not exceed agency policy or the limit indicated in the medical record.	

SKILL 35-2

Administering a Tube Feeding *(Continued)*

Excellent	Satisfactory	Needs Practice		Comments
——	——	——	14. Flush tube with 30 mL of water for irrigation. Disconnect syringe from tubing and cap end of tubing while preparing the formula feeding equipment. Remove gloves.	
——	——	——	15. Put on gloves before preparing, assembling, and handling any part of the feeding system.	
——	——	——	16. Administer feeding.	
			When Using a Feeding Bag (Open System)	
——	——	——	a. Label the bag and/or tubing with date and time. Hang the bag on an IV pole and adjust to about 12 inches above the stomach. Clamp the tubing.	
——	——	——	b. Check the expiration date of the formula. Cleanse the top of the feeding container with a disinfectant before opening it. Pour the formula into the feeding bag and allow the solution to run through the tubing. Close the clamp.	
——	——	——	c. Attach the feeding setup to the feeding tube, open the clamp, and regulate the drip according to the medical order, or allow the feeding to run in over 30 minutes.	
——	——	——	d. *Add 30 to 60 mL (1 to 2 oz) of water for irrigation to the feeding bag when the feeding is almost completed and allow it to run through the tube.*	
——	——	——	e. Clamp the tubing immediately after water has been instilled. Disconnect the feeding setup from the feeding tube. Clamp the tube and cover the end with the cap.	
			When Using a Large Syringe (Open System)	
——	——	——	a. Remove the plunger from a 30- or 60-mL syringe.	
——	——	——	b. Attach a syringe to the feeding tube, pour a premeasured amount of tube feeding formula into the syringe, open the clamp, and allow the food to enter the tube. Regulate the rate, fast or slow, by height of the syringe. *Do not push formula with syringe plunger.*	
——	——	——	c. *Add 30 to 60 mL (1 to 2 oz) of water for irrigation to the syringe when feeding is almost completed, and allow it to run through the tube.*	
——	——	——	d. When the syringe has emptied, hold the syringe high and disconnect it from tube. Clamp the tube and cover the end with the cap.	

SKILL 35-2
Administering a Tube Feeding *(Continued)*

Excellent	Satisfactory	Needs Practice		Comments

When Using an Enteral Feeding Pump

a. Close the flow-regulator clamp on the tubing and fill the feeding bag with prescribed formula. Amount used depends on agency policy. Place a label on the container with the patient's name, date, and time the feeding was hung.

b. Hang the feeding container on an IV pole. Allow the solution to flow through the tubing.

c. Connect to the feeding pump following the manufacturer's directions. Set the rate. Maintain the patient in the upright position throughout the feeding. If the patient needs to temporarily lie flat, pause the feeding. Resume the feeding after the patient's position has been changed back to at least 30 to 45 degrees.

d. *Check placement of the tube and gastric residual every 4 to 6 hours.*

17. Observe the patient's response during and after tube feeding and assess the abdomen at least once per shift.

18. *Have the patient remain in the upright position for at least 1 hour after feeding.*

19. Remove equipment and return the patient to a position of comfort. Remove gloves. Raise the side rail and lower the bed.

20. Put on gloves. Wash and clean equipment or replace according to agency policy. Remove gloves.

21. Remove additional PPE, if used. Perform hand hygiene.

Skill Checklists for Fundamentals of Nursing:
The Art and Science of Person-Centered Nursing Care, 8th edition

Name _____   Date _____

Unit _____   Position _____

Instructor/Evaluator: _____   Position _____

Excellent	Satisfactory	Needs Practice	SKILL 35-3 **Removing a Nasogastric Tube**	Comments
			Goal: The tube is removed with minimal discomfort to the patient, and the patient maintains an adequate nutritional intake.	
___	___	___	1. Check the medical record for the order for removal of the NG tube.	
___	___	___	2. Perform hand hygiene and put on PPE, if indicated.	
___	___	___	3. Identify the patient.	
___	___	___	4. Explain the procedure to the patient and why this intervention is warranted. Describe that it will entail a quick few moments of discomfort. Perform key abdominal assessments.	
___	___	___	5. Pull the patient's bedside curtain. Raise the bed to a comfortable working position, usually elbow height of the caregiver. Assist the patient into a 30- to 45-degree position. Place a towel or disposable pad across the patient's chest. Give tissues and the emesis basin to the patient.	
___	___	___	6. Put on gloves. Discontinue suction and separate the tube from the suction. Unpin the tube from the patient's gown and carefully remove the adhesive tape from the patient's nose.	
___	___	___	7. Check placement and attach syringe and *flush with 10 mL of water or normal saline solution (optional) or clear with 30 to 50 mL of air.*	
___	___	___	8. Clamp tube with fingers by doubling tube on itself. *Instruct the patient to take a deep breath and hold it. Quickly and carefully remove the tube while the patient holds breath.* Coil the tube in the disposable pad as you remove it from the patient.	
___	___	___	9. Dispose of the tube per facility policy. Remove gloves. Perform hand hygiene.	
___	___	___	10. Offer mouth care to the patient and facial tissue to blow the nose. Lower the bed and assist the patient to a position of comfort as needed.	
___	___	___	11. Remove equipment, and raise the side rail and the lower bed.	

Removing a Nasogastric Tube *(Continued)*

Excellent	Satisfactory	Needs Practice		Comments
——	——	——	12. Put on gloves and measure the amount of nasogastric drainage in the collection device. Record the measurement on the output flow record, subtracting irrigant fluids if necessary. Add a solidifying agent to the nasogastric drainage and dispose of the drainage according to facility policy.	
——	——	——	13. Remove additional PPE, if used. Perform hand hygiene.	

Skill Checklists for Fundamentals of Nursing:
The Art and Science of Person-Centered Nursing Care, 8th edition

Name _____   Date _____

Unit _____   Position _____

Instructor/Evaluator: _____   Position _____

Excellent	Satisfactory	Needs Practice	SKILL 35-4 **Obtaining a Capillary Blood Sample for Glucose Testing**	
			Goal: Patient blood glucose levels are accurately monitored.	**Comments**
⎯ ⎯ ⎯			1. Check the patient's medical record or nursing plan of care for the monitoring schedule. You may decide that additional testing is indicated based on nursing judgment and the patient's condition.	
⎯ ⎯ ⎯			2. Gather equipment. Check the expiration date on the blood test strips.	
⎯ ⎯ ⎯			3. Perform hand hygiene and put on PPE, if indicated.	
⎯ ⎯ ⎯			4. Identify the patient. Explain the procedure to the patient and instruct the patient about the need for monitoring blood glucose.	
⎯ ⎯ ⎯			5. Close the curtains around the bed and close the door to the room, if possible.	
⎯ ⎯ ⎯			6. Turn on the monitor.	
⎯ ⎯ ⎯			7. Enter the patient's identification number or scan the patient's identification bracelet, if required, according to facility policy.	
⎯ ⎯ ⎯			8. Put on nonsterile gloves.	
⎯ ⎯ ⎯			9. Prepare the lancet using aseptic technique.	
⎯ ⎯ ⎯			10. Remove the test strip from the vial. *Recap the container immediately.* Test strips also come individually wrapped. *Check that the code number for the strip matches the code number on the monitor screen.*	
⎯ ⎯ ⎯			11. Insert the strip into the meter according to directions for that specific device. Alternately, the strip may be placed in the meter after collection of a sample on the test strip, depending on meter in use.	
⎯ ⎯ ⎯			12. *Have the patient wash hands with skin cleanser and warm water and dry thoroughly. Alternately, cleanse the skin with an alcohol swab. Allow skin to dry completely.*	
⎯ ⎯ ⎯			13. Choose a skin site free of lesions and calluses. Make sure there is no edema, and that the site is warm.	
⎯ ⎯ ⎯			14. Hold the lancet perpendicular to the skin and pierce the site with the lancet.	

Obtaining a Capillary Blood Sample for Glucose Testing (Continued)

Excellent	Satisfactory	Needs Practice		Comments
——	——	——	15. Wipe away the first drop of blood with a gauze square or cotton ball if recommended by the manufacturer of the monitor.	
——	——	——	16. Encourage bleeding by lowering the hand, making use of gravity. Lightly stroke the finger, if necessary, until a sufficient amount of blood has formed to cover the sample area on the strip, based on monitor requirements (check instructions for the monitor). Take care not to squeeze the finger, not to squeeze at the puncture site, or not to touch the puncture site or blood.	
——	——	——	17. Gently touch a drop of blood to the pad to the test strip without smearing it. Depending on the meter in use, insert the strip in the meter after collection of the sample on the test strip.	
——	——	——	18. Press the time button if directed by the manufacturer.	
——	——	——	19. Apply pressure to the puncture site with a cotton ball or dry gauze. *Do not use an alcohol wipe.*	
——	——	——	20. Read the blood glucose results and document appropriately at bedside. Inform the patient of the test result.	
——	——	——	21. Turn off the meter, remove the test strip, and dispose of supplies appropriately. Place the lancet in a sharps container.	
——	——	——	22. Remove gloves and any other PPE, if used. Perform hand hygiene.	

Skill Checklists for Fundamentals of Nursing:
The Art and Science of Person-Centered Nursing Care, 8th edition

Name _____   Date _____

Unit _____   Position _____

Instructor/Evaluator: _____   Position _____

SKILL 36-1

Assessing Bladder Volume Using an Ultrasound Bladder Scanner

Goal: The volume of urine in the bladder is accurately measured.

Excellent	Satisfactory	Needs Practice		Comments
——	——	——	1. Review the patient's medical record for any limitations in physical activity. Gather equipment.	
——	——	——	2. Perform hand hygiene and put on PPE, if indicated.	
——	——	——	3. Identify the patient.	
——	——	——	4. Close the curtains around the bed and close the door to the room, if possible. Discuss the procedure with the patient and assess the patient's ability to assist with the procedure, as well as personal hygiene preferences.	
——	——	——	5. Adjust the bed to a comfortable working height; usually elbow height of the caregiver. Place the patient in a supine position. Drape patient. Stand on the patient's right side if you are right-handed, patient's left side if you are left-handed.	
——	——	——	6. Put on clean gloves.	
——	——	——	7. Press the ON button. Wait until the device warms up. Press the SCAN button to turn on the scanning screen.	
——	——	——	8. Press the appropriate gender button. The appropriate icon for male or female will appear on the screen.	
——	——	——	9. Clean the scanner head with the appropriate cleaner.	
——	——	——	10. Gently palpate the patient's symphysis pubis (anterior midline junction of pubic bones). Place a generous amount of ultrasound gel or gel pad midline on the patient's abdomen, about 1 to 1.5 inches above the symphysis pubis.	
——	——	——	11. Place the scanner head on the gel or gel pad, *with the directional icon on the scanner head toward the patient's head. Aim the scanner head toward the bladder (point the scanner head slightly downward toward the coccyx).* Press and release the scan button.	
——	——	——	12. Observe the image on the scanner screen. *Adjust the scanner head to center the bladder image on the crossbars.*	
——	——	——	13. Press and hold the DONE button until it beeps. Read the volume measurement on the screen. Print the results, if required, by pressing PRINT.	

Assessing Bladder Volume Using an Ultrasound Bladder Scanner *(Continued)*

Excellent	Satisfactory	Needs Practice		Comments
——	——	——	14. Use a washcloth or paper towel to remove remaining gel from the patient's skin. Alternately, gently remove gel pad from patient's skin. Return the patient to a comfortable position. Remove your gloves and ensure that the patient is covered.	
——	——	——	15. Lower bed height and adjust head of bed to a comfortable position. Reattach call bell, if necessary.	
——	——	——	16. Remove additional PPE, if used. Perform hand hygiene.	

Skill Checklists for Fundamentals of Nursing:
The Art and Science of Person-Centered Nursing Care, 8th edition

Name _____   Date _____

Unit _____   Position _____

Instructor/Evaluator: _____   Position _____

Excellent	Satisfactory	Needs Practice	SKILL 36-2 **Assisting With the Use of a Bedpan**	Comments
			Goal: The patient is able to void with assistance.	
——	——	——	1. Review the patient's medical record for any limitations in physical activity. Gather equipment.	
——	——	——	2. Perform hand hygiene and put on PPE, if indicated.	
——	——	——	3. Identify the patient.	
——	——	——	4. Assemble equipment on the chair next to the bed within reach.	
——	——	——	5. Close curtains around the bed and close the door to the room, if possible. Discuss the procedure with the patient and assess the patient's ability to assist with the procedure, as well as personal hygiene preferences.	
——	——	——	6. Unless contraindicated, apply powder to the rim of the bedpan. Place bedpan and cover on the chair next to the bed. Put on gloves.	
——	——	——	7. Adjust bed to comfortable working height, usually elbow height of the caregiver. Place the patient in a supine position, with the head of the bed elevated about 30 degrees, unless contraindicated.	
——	——	——	8. Fold the top linen back just enough to allow placement of the bedpan. If there is no waterproof pad on the bed and time allows, consider placing a waterproof pad under the patient's buttocks before placing the bedpan.	
——	——	——	9. Ask the patient to bend the knees. Have the patient lift the hips upward. Assist the patient, if necessary, by placing your hand that is closest to the patient palm up, under the lower back, and assist with lifting. Slip the bedpan into place with the other hand.	
——	——	——	10. *Ensure that the bedpan is in proper position and the patient's buttocks are resting on the rounded shelf of the regular bedpan or the shallow rim of the fracture bedpan.*	
——	——	——	11. Raise the head of the bed as near to sitting position as tolerated, unless contraindicated. Cover the patient with bed linens.	
——	——	——	12. *Place the call bell and toilet tissue within easy reach. Place the bed in the lowest position.* Leave the patient if it is safe to do so. Use side rails appropriately.	

Excellent	Satisfactory	Needs Practice	SKILL 36-2 **Assisting With the Use of a Bedpan** *(Continued)*	
				Comments
——	——	——	13. Remove gloves and additional PPE, if used. Perform hand hygiene.	
			Removing the Bedpan	
——	——	——	14. Perform hand hygiene and put on gloves and additional PPE, as indicated. Adjust the bed to a comfortable working height, usually elbow height of the caregiver. Have a receptacle, such as a plastic trash bag, handy for discarding tissue.	
——	——	——	15. Lower the head of the bed, if necessary, to about 30 degrees. Remove the bedpan in the same manner in which it was offered, being careful to hold it steady. Ask the patient to bend the knees and lift the buttocks up from the bedpan. Assist the patient, if necessary, by placing your hand that is closest to the patient palm up, under the lower back, and assist with lifting. Place the bedpan on the bed-side chair and cover it.	
——	——	——	16. If the patient needs assistance with hygiene, wrap tissue around the hand several times, and wipe the patient clean, using one stroke from the pubic area toward the anal area. Discard tissue. Use warm, moist, disposable washcloth and skin cleanser to clean perineal area. Place the patient on his or her side and spread buttocks to clean the anal area.	
——	——	——	17. Do not place toilet tissue in the bedpan if a specimen is required or if output is being recorded. Place toilet tissue in the appropriate receptacle.	
——	——	——	18. Return the patient to a comfortable position. Make sure the linens under the patient are dry. Replace or remove pad under the patient, as necessary. Remove your gloves and ensure that the patient is covered.	
——	——	——	19. Raise the side rail. Lower the bed height and adjust the head of the bed to a comfortable position. Reattach the call bell.	
——	——	——	20. Offer patient supplies to wash and dry the hands, assisting as necessary.	
——	——	——	21. Put on clean gloves. Empty and clean the bedpan, measuring the urine in a graduated container, as necessary. Discard trash receptacle with used toilet paper per facility policy.	
——	——	——	22. Remove additional PPE, if used. Perform hand hygiene.	

Skill Checklists for Fundamentals of Nursing:
The Art and Science of Person-Centered Nursing Care, 8th edition

Name _____   Date _____

Unit _____   Position _____

Instructor/Evaluator: _____   Position _____

SKILL 36-3
Assisting With the Use of a Urinal

Excellent	Satisfactory	Needs Practice	**Goal:** The patient is able to void with assistance.	Comments
___	___	___	1. Review the patient's medical record for any limitations in physical activity. Gather equipment.	
___	___	___	2. Perform hand hygiene and put on PPE, if indicated.	
___	___	___	3. Identify the patient.	
___	___	___	4. Assemble equipment on the chair next to the bed within reach.	
___	___	___	5. Close the curtains around the bed and close the door to the room, if possible. Discuss the procedure with the patient and assess the patient's ability to assist with the procedure, as well as personal hygiene preferences.	
___	___	___	6. Put on gloves.	
___	___	___	7. Assist the patient to an appropriate position, as necessary: standing at the bedside, lying on one side or back, sitting in bed with the head elevated, or sitting on the side of the bed.	
___	___	___	8. If the patient remains in the bed, fold the linens just enough to allow for proper placement of the urinal.	
___	___	___	9. If the patient is not standing, have him spread his legs slightly. *Hold the urinal close to the penis and position the penis completely within the urinal. Keep the bottom of the urinal lower than the penis. If necessary, assist the patient to hold the urinal in place.*	
___	___	___	10. Cover the patient with the bed linens.	
___	___	___	11. Place the call bell and toilet tissue within easy reach. Have a receptacle, such as a plastic trash bag, handy for discarding tissue. Ensure that the bed is in the lowest position. Leave the patient if it is safe to do so. Use the side rails appropriately.	
___	___	___	12. Remove gloves and additional PPE, if used. Perform hand hygiene.	
			Removing the Urinal	
___	___	___	13. Perform hand hygiene. Put on gloves and additional PPE, as indicated.	

SKILL 36-3

Assisting With the Use of a Urinal *(Continued)*

Excellent	Satisfactory	Needs Practice		Comments
——	——	——	14. Pull back the patient's bed linens just enough to remove the urinal. Remove the urinal. Cover the open end of the urinal. Place on the bedside chair. If patient needs assistance with hygiene, wrap tissue around the hand several times, and wipe patient dry. Place tissue in receptacle. Use warm, moist, disposable washcloth and skin cleanser to clean perineal area as necessary, and as per patient request.	
——	——	——	15. Return the patient to a comfortable position. Make sure the linens under the patient are dry. Remove your gloves and ensure that the patient is covered.	
——	——	——	16. Ensure that the patient call bell is in reach.	
——	——	——	17. Offer the patient supplies to wash and dry his hands, assisting as necessary.	
——	——	——	18. Put on clean gloves. Empty and clean the urinal, measuring the urine in a graduated container, as necessary. Discard the trash receptacle with used toilet paper per facility policy.	
——	——	——	19. Remove gloves and additional PPE, if used, and perform hand hygiene.	

Skill Checklists for Fundamentals of Nursing:
The Art and Science of Person-Centered Nursing Care, 8th edition

Name _____   Date _____

Unit _____   Position _____

Instructor/Evaluator: _____   Position _____

SKILL 36-4

Applying an External Condom Catheter

Goal: The patient's urinary elimination will be maintained, with a urine output of at least 30 mL/hour, and the bladder is not distended.

Excellent	Satisfactory	Needs Practice		Comments
——	——	——	1. Gather equipment.	
——	——	——	2. Perform hand hygiene and put on PPE, if indicated.	
——	——	——	3. Identify the patient.	
——	——	——	4. Close curtains around the bed and close the door to the room, if possible. Discuss the procedure with the patient. Ask the patient if he has any allergies, especially to latex.	
——	——	——	5. Assemble equipment on the overbed table within reach.	
——	——	——	6. Adjust the bed to a comfortable working height, usually elbow height of the caregiver. Stand on the patient's right side if you are right-handed, or on patient's left side if you are left-handed.	
——	——	——	7. Prepare the urinary drainage setup or reusable leg bag for attachment to the condom sheath.	
——	——	——	8. Position the patient on his back with thighs slightly apart. Drape the patient so that only the area around the penis is exposed. Slide a waterproof pad under the patient.	
——	——	——	9. Put on disposable gloves. Trim any long pubic hair that is in contact with the penis.	
——	——	——	10. Clean the genital area with a washcloth, skin cleanser, and warm water. If the patient is uncircumcised, retract the foreskin and clean the glans of the penis. Replace the foreskin. Clean the tip of the penis first, moving the washcloth in a circular motion from the meatus outward. Wash the shaft of the penis using downward strokes toward the pubic area. Rinse and dry. Remove gloves. Perform hand hygiene again.	
——	——	——	11. Apply skin protectant to the penis and allow to dry.	
——	——	——	12. Roll the condom sheath outward onto itself. Grasp the penis firmly with your nondominant hand. *Apply the condom sheath by rolling it onto the penis with your dominant hand. Leave 1 to 2 inches (2.5 to 5 cm) of space between the tip of the penis and the end of the condom sheath.*	

Applying an External Condom Catheter *(Continued)*

Excellent	Satisfactory	Needs Practice		Comments
——	——	——	13. *Apply pressure to the sheath at the base of the penis for 10 to 15 seconds.*	
——	——	——	14. Connect the condom sheath to the drainage setup. Avoid kinking or twisting the drainage tubing.	
——	——	——	15. Remove gloves. Secure drainage tubing to the patient's inner thigh with a Velcro leg strap or tape. Leave some slack in the tubing for leg movement.	
——	——	——	16. Assist the patient to a comfortable position. Cover the patient with bed linens. Place the bed in the lowest position.	
——	——	——	17. Secure the drainage bag below the level of the bladder. Check that drainage tubing is not kinked and that movement of the side rails does not interfere with the drainage bag.	
——	——	——	18. Remove equipment. Remove gloves and additional PPE, if used. Perform hand hygiene.	

Skill Checklists for Fundamentals of Nursing:
The Art and Science of Person-Centered Nursing Care, 8th edition

Name _____   Date _____

Unit _____   Position _____

Instructor/Evaluator: _____   Position _____

SKILL 36-5
Catheterizing the Female Urinary Bladder

Goal: The patient's urinary elimination is maintained, with a urine output of at least 30 mL/hour, and the patient's bladder is not distended.

Excellent	Satisfactory	Needs Practice		Comments
___	___	___	1. Review the patient's chart for any limitations in physical activity. Confirm the medical order for indwelling catheter insertion.	
___	___	___	2. Gather equipment. Obtain assistance from another staff member, if necessary.	
___	___	___	3. Perform hand hygiene and put on PPE, if indicated.	
___	___	___	4. Identify the patient.	
___	___	___	5. Close curtains around the bed and close the door to the room, if possible. Discuss the procedure with the patient and assess the patient's ability to assist with the procedure. Ask the patient if she has any allergies, especially to latex or iodine.	
___	___	___	6. Provide good lighting. Artificial light is recommended (use of a flashlight requires an assistant to hold and position it). Place a trash receptacle within easy reach.	
___	___	___	7. Assemble equipment on the overbed table within reach.	
___	___	___	8. Adjust the bed to a comfortable working height, usually elbow height of the caregiver. Stand on the patient's right side if you are right-handed, on the patient's left side if you are left-handed.	
___	___	___	9. Assist the patient to a dorsal recumbent position with knees flexed, feet about 2 feet apart, with her legs abducted. Drape the patient. Alternately, the Sims', or lateral, position can be used. Place the patient's buttocks near the edge of the bed with her shoulders at the opposite edge and her knees drawn toward her chest. Allow the patient to lie on either side, depending on which position is easiest for the nurse and best for the patient's comfort. Slide a waterproof pad under the patient.	
___	___	___	10. Put on clean gloves. Clean the perineal area with a washcloth, skin cleanser, and warm water, using a different corner of the washcloth with each stroke. Wipe from above the orifice downward toward sacrum (front to back). Rinse and dry. Remove gloves. Perform hand hygiene again.	

SKILL 36-5

Catheterizing the Female Urinary Bladder *(Continued)*

Excellent	Satisfactory	Needs Practice		Comments
⎯	⎯	⎯	11. Prepare a urine drainage setup if a separate urine collection system is to be used. Secure to the bed frame according to the manufacturer's directions.	
⎯	⎯	⎯	12. Open sterile catheterization tray on a clean overbed table using sterile technique.	
⎯	⎯	⎯	13. Put on sterile gloves. Grasp the upper corners of the drape and unfold the drape without touching nonsterile areas. Fold back a corner on each side to make a cuff over gloved hands. Ask the patient to lift her buttocks and slide a sterile drape under her with gloves protected by the cuff.	
⎯	⎯	⎯	14. Based on facility policy, position the fenestrated sterile drape. Place a fenestrated sterile drape over the perineal area, exposing the labia. (*Note:* the fenestrated drape is not shown in the remaining illustrations in order to provide a clear view of the procedure.)	
⎯	⎯	⎯	15. Place a sterile tray on the drape between the patient's thighs.	
⎯	⎯	⎯	16. Open all the supplies. Open a package of antiseptic swabs. Alternately, fluff cotton balls in the tray before pouring antiseptic solution over them. Open a specimen container if a specimen is to be obtained.	
⎯	⎯	⎯	17. Lubricate 1 to 2 inches of catheter tip.	
⎯	⎯	⎯	18. With thumb and one finger of your nondominant hand, spread the labia and identify the meatus. *Be prepared to maintain separation of the labia with one hand until the catheter is inserted and urine is flowing well and continuously.* If the patient is in the side-lying position, lift the upper buttock and labia to expose the urinary meatus.	
⎯	⎯	⎯	19. Use your dominant hand to pick up an antiseptic swab or use forceps to pick up a cotton ball. *Clean one labial fold, top to bottom (from above the meatus down toward the rectum), then discard the cotton ball. Using a new cotton ball/swab for each stroke, continue to clean the other labial fold, then directly over the meatus.*	
⎯	⎯	⎯	20. With your noncontaminated, dominant hand, place the drainage end of the catheter in receptacle. If the catheter is pre-attached to sterile tubing and a drainage container (closed drainage system), position the catheter and setup within easy reach on the sterile field. Ensure that the clamp on the drainage bag is closed.	

Catheterizing the Female Urinary Bladder *(Continued)*

Excellent	Satisfactory	Needs Practice		Comments
—	—	—	21. *Using your dominant hand, hold the catheter 2 to 3 inches from the tip and insert slowly into the urethra. Advance the catheter until there is a return of urine—approximately 2 to 3 inches (4.8 to 7.2 cm). Once urine drains, advance the catheter another 2 to 3 inches (4.8 to 7.2 cm). Do not force the catheter through the urethra into the bladder.* Ask the patient to breathe deeply, and rotate the catheter gently if slight resistance is met as the catheter reaches the external sphincter.	
—	—	—	22. Hold the catheter securely at the meatus with your non-dominant hand. Use your dominant hand to inflate the catheter balloon. Inject the entire volume of sterile water supplied in the prefilled syringe.	
—	—	—	23. Pull gently on the catheter after the balloon is inflated to feel resistance.	
—	—	—	24. Attach the catheter to the drainage system if not already preattached.	
—	—	—	25. Remove equipment and dispose of it according to facility policy. Discard the syringe in a sharps container. Wash and dry the perineal area, as needed.	
—	—	—	26. Remove gloves. *Secure the catheter tubing to the patient's inner thigh with a Velcro® leg strap, catheter securing device, or tape.* Leave some slack in catheter for leg movement.	
—	—	—	27. Assist the patient to a comfortable position. Cover the patient with bed linens. Place the bed in the lowest position.	
—	—	—	28. Secure the drainage bag below the level of the bladder. Check that the drainage tubing is not kinked and that movement of the side rails does not interfere with the catheter or drainage bag.	
—	—	—	29. Put on clean gloves. Obtain urine specimen immediately, if needed, from the drainage bag. Label the specimen. Send the urine specimen to the laboratory promptly or refrigerate it.	
—	—	—	30. Remove gloves and additional PPE, if used. Perform hand hygiene.	

Skill Checklists for Fundamentals of Nursing:
The Art and Science of Person-Centered Nursing Care, 8th edition

Name _____ Date _____

Unit _____ Position _____

Instructor/Evaluator: _____ Position _____

SKILL 36-6
Catheterizing the Male Urinary Bladder

Goal: The patient's urinary elimination is maintained, with a urine output of at least 30 mL/hour, and the patient's bladder is not distended.

Excellent	Satisfactory	Needs Practice		Comments
―	―	―	1. Review chart for any limitations in physical activity. Confirm the medical order for indwelling catheter insertion.	
―	―	―	2. Gather equipment. Obtain assistance from another staff member, if necessary.	
―	―	―	3. Perform hand hygiene and put on PPE, if indicated.	
―	―	―	4. Identify the patient.	
―	―	―	5. Close curtains around the bed and close the door to the room, if possible. Discuss the procedure with the patient and assess the patient's ability to assist with the procedure. Ask the patient if he has any allergies, especially to latex or iodine.	
―	―	―	6. Provide good lighting. Artificial light is recommended (use of a flashlight requires an assistant to hold and position it). Place a trash receptacle within easy reach.	
―	―	―	7. Assemble equipment on the overbed table within reach.	
―	―	―	8. Adjust the bed to a comfortable working height, usually elbow height of the caregiver. Stand on the patient's right side if you are right-handed, on the patient's left side if you are left-handed.	
―	―	―	9. Position the patient on his back with thighs slightly apart. Drape the patient so that only the area around the penis is exposed. Slide a waterproof pad under the patient.	
―	―	―	10. Put on clean gloves. Clean the genital area with a washcloth, skin cleanser, and warm water. Clean the tip of the penis first, moving the washcloth in a circular motion from the meatus outward. Wash the shaft of the penis using downward strokes toward the pubic area. Rinse and dry. Remove gloves. Perform hand hygiene again.	
―	―	―	11. Prepare a urine drainage setup if a separate urine collection system is to be used. Secure to the bed frame according to the manufacturer's directions.	
―	―	―	12. Open the sterile catheterization tray on a clean overbed table, using sterile technique.	

SKILL 36-6
Catheterizing the Male Urinary Bladder *(Continued)*

Excellent	Satisfactory	Needs Practice		Comments
——	——	——	13. Put on sterile gloves. Open a sterile drape and place on the patient's thighs. Place the fenestrated drape with the opening over the penis.	
——	——	——	14. Place the catheter set on or next to the patient's legs on a sterile drape.	
——	——	——	15. Open all the supplies. Open a package of antiseptic swabs. Alternately, fluff cotton balls in the tray before pouring antiseptic solution over them. Open a specimen container if a specimen is to be obtained. Remove the cap from a syringe prefilled with lubricant.	
——	——	——	16. Place the drainage end of the catheter in the receptacle. If the catheter is pre-attached to the sterile tubing and drainage container (closed drainage system), position the catheter and setup within easy reach on a sterile field. Ensure that the clamp on the drainage bag is closed.	
——	——	——	17. Lift the penis with your nondominant hand. Retract the foreskin in the uncircumcised patient. *Be prepared to keep this hand in this position until the catheter is inserted and urine is flowing well and continuously. Use your dominant hand to pick up an antiseptic swab or use forceps to pick up a cotton ball. Using a circular motion, clean the penis, moving from the meatus down the glans of the penis. Repeat this cleansing motion two more times, using a new cotton ball/swab each time. Discard each cotton ball/swab after one use.*	
——	——	——	18. Hold the penis with a slight upward tension and perpendicular to the patient's body. Use the dominant hand to pick up the lubricant syringe. *Gently insert the tip of the syringe with lubricant into the urethra and instill the 10 mL of lubricant.*	
——	——	——	19. Use your dominant hand to pick up the catheter and hold it an inch or two from the tip. Ask the patient to bear down as if voiding. *Insert catheter tip into meatus. Ask the patient to take deep breaths. Advance the catheter to the bifurcation or "Y" level of the ports. Do not use force to introduce the catheter.* If the catheter resists entry, ask the patient to breathe deeply and rotate the catheter slightly.	
——	——	——	20. Hold the catheter securely at the meatus with your nondominant hand. Use your dominant hand to inflate the catheter balloon. *Inject the entire volume of sterile water supplied in the prefilled syringe. Once the balloon is inflated, the catheter may be gently pulled back into place. Replace the foreskin over the catheter.* Lower the penis.	

SKILL 36-6

Catheterizing the Male Urinary Bladder *(Continued)*

Excellent	Satisfactory	Needs Practice		Comments
——	——	——	21. Pull gently on the catheter after the balloon is inflated to feel resistance.	
——	——	——	22. Attach the catheter to the drainage system, if necessary.	
——	——	——	23. Remove equipment and dispose of it according to facility policy. Discard the syringe in a sharps container. Wash and dry the perineal area as needed.	
——	——	——	24. Remove gloves. Secure the catheter tubing to the patient's inner thigh or lower abdomen (with the penis directed toward the patient's chest) with a Velcro® leg strap, catheter securing device, or tape. Leave some slack in the catheter for leg movement.	
——	——	——	25. Assist the patient to a comfortable position. Cover the patient with bed linens. Place the bed in the lowest position.	
——	——	——	26. Secure the drainage bag below the level of the bladder. Check that the drainage tubing is not kinked and that movement of the side rails does not interfere with the catheter or drainage bag.	
——	——	——	27. Put on clean gloves. Obtain a urine specimen immediately, if needed, from the drainage bag. Label the specimen. Send the urine specimen to the laboratory promptly or refrigerate it.	
——	——	——	28. Remove gloves and additional PPE, if used. Perform hand hygiene.	

Skill Checklists for Fundamentals of Nursing:
The Art and Science of Person-Centered Nursing Care, 8th edition

Name _____ Date _____

Unit _____ Position _____

Instructor/Evaluator: _____ Position _____

Excellent	Satisfactory	Needs Practice	SKILL 36-7 **Performing Intermittent Closed Catheter Irrigation**	Comments
			Goal: The patient exhibits the free flow of urine through the catheter.	
____ ____ ____			1. Confirm the order for catheter irrigation in the medical record.	
____ ____ ____			2. Gather equipment.	
____ ____ ____			3. Perform hand hygiene and put on PPE, if indicated.	
____ ____ ____			4. Identify the patient.	
			5. Close curtains around the bed and close the door to the room, if possible. Discuss the procedure with the patient.	
____ ____ ____			6. Assemble equipment on the overbed table within reach.	
____ ____ ____			7. Adjust the bed to a comfortable working height, usually elbow height of the caregiver.	
____ ____ ____			8. Put on gloves. Empty the catheter drainage bag and measure the amount of urine, noting the amount and characteristics of the urine. Remove gloves.	
____ ____ ____			9. Assist patient to a comfortable position and expose the access port on the catheter setup. Place a waterproof pad under the catheter and aspiration port. Remove the catheter from the device or tape the anchoring catheter to the patient.	
____ ____ ____			10. Open supplies, using aseptic technique. Pour the sterile solution into a sterile basin. Aspirate the prescribed amount of irrigant (usually 30 to 60 mL) into sterile syringe. Put on gloves.	
____ ____ ____			11. *Cleanse the access port on the catheter with antimicrobial swab.*	
____ ____ ____			12. Clamp or fold the catheter tubing below the access port.	
____ ____ ____			13. Attach the syringe to the access port on the catheter using a twisting motion. *Gently instill solution into the catheter.*	
____ ____ ____			14. Remove the syringe from the access port. *Unclamp or unfold tubing and allow irrigant and urine to flow into the drainage bag.* Repeat procedure, as necessary.	

Excellent	Satisfactory	Needs Practice		
			SKILL 36-7 **Performing Intermittent Closed Catheter Irrigation** *(Continued)*	
				Comments
——	——	——	15. Remove gloves. Secure catheter tubing to the patient's inner thigh or lower abdomen (if a male patient) with anchoring device or tape. Leave some slack in the catheter for leg movement.	
——	——	——	16. Assist the patient to a comfortable position. Cover the patient with bed linens. Place the bed in the lowest position.	
——	——	——	17. Secure drainage bag below the level of the bladder. Check that drainage tubing is not kinked and that movement of the side rails does not interfere with the catheter or drainage bag.	
——	——	——	18. Remove equipment and discard syringe in appropriate receptacle. Remove gloves and additional PPE, if used. Perform hand hygiene.	
——	——	——	19. Assess the patient's response to the procedure and the quality and amount of drainage after the irrigation.	

Skill Checklists for Fundamentals of Nursing:
The Art and Science of Person-Centered Nursing Care, 8th edition

Name _____   Date _____

Unit _____   Position _____

Instructor/Evaluator: _____   Position _____

Excellent	Satisfactory	Needs Practice	SKILL 36-8 **Administering a Continuous Closed Bladder or Catheter Irrigation**	
			Goal: The patient exhibits free-flowing urine through the catheter.	**Comments**
____	____	____	1. Confirm the order for catheter irrigation in the medical record, including infusion parameters. If irrigation is to be implemented via gravity infusion, calculate the drip rate. Often, orders are to infuse to keep the urine clear of blood.	
____	____	____	2. Gather equipment.	
____	____	____	3. Perform hand hygiene and put on PPE, if indicated.	
____	____	____	4. Identify the patient.	
____	____	____	5. Close the curtains around the bed and close the door to the room, if possible. Discuss the procedure with the patient.	
____	____	____	6. Assemble equipment on the overbed table within reach.	
____	____	____	7. Adjust the bed to a comfortable working height, usually elbow height of the caregiver.	
____	____	____	8. Empty the catheter drainage bag and measure the amount of urine, noting the amount and characteristics of the urine.	
____	____	____	9. Assist the patient to a comfortable position and expose the irrigation port on the catheter setup. Place a waterproof pad under the catheter and aspiration port.	
____	____	____	10. Prepare a sterile irrigation bag for use as directed by the manufacturer. Clearly label the solution as "Bladder Irrigant." Include the date and time on the label. Hang bag on an IV pole 2.5 to 3 feet above the level of the patient's bladder. Secure the tubing clamp and insert the sterile tubing with drip chamber to the container using aseptic technique. Release the clamp and remove the protective cover on the end of the tubing without contaminating it. Allow the solution to flush the tubing and remove air. Clamp the tubing and replace the end cover.	
____	____	____	11. Put on gloves. *Cleanse the irrigation port on the catheter with an alcohol swab. Using aseptic technique, attach irrigation tubing to the irrigation port of the three-way indwelling catheter.*	
____	____	____	12. Check the drainage tubing to make sure clamp, if present, is open.	

SKILL 36-8

Administering a Continuous Closed Bladder or Catheter Irrigation *(Continued)*

Excellent	Satisfactory	Needs Practice		Comments
——	——	——	13. *Release the clamp on the irrigation tubing and regulate the flow at the determined drip rate, according to the ordered rate.* If the bladder irrigation is to be done with a medicated solution, use an electronic infusion device to regulate the flow.	
——	——	——	14. Remove gloves. Assist the patient to a comfortable position. Cover the patient with bed linens. Place the bed in the lowest position.	
——	——	——	15. Assess the patient's response to the procedure, and quality and amount of drainage.	
——	——	——	16. Remove equipment. Remove gloves and additional PPE, if used. Perform hand hygiene.	
——	——	——	17. As irrigation fluid container nears empty, clamp the administration tubing. Do not allow the drip chamber to empty. Disconnect the empty bag and attach a new full irrigation solution bag.	
——	——	——	18. Put on gloves and empty drainage collection bag as each new container is hung and recorded.	

Skill Checklists for Fundamentals of Nursing:
The Art and Science of Person-Centered Nursing Care, 8th edition

Name _____   Date _____

Unit _____   Position _____

Instructor/Evaluator: _____   Position _____

Excellent	Satisfactory	Needs Practice	SKILL 36-9 **Emptying and Changing a Stoma Appliance** **on an Ileal Conduit**	
			Goal: The stoma appliance is applied correctly to the skin to allow urine to drain freely.	**Comments**
____	____	____	1. Gather equipment.	
____	____	____	2. Perform hand hygiene and put on PPE, if indicated.	
____	____	____	3. Identify the patient.	
____	____	____	4. Close the curtains around the bed and close the door to the room, if possible. Explain what you are going to do and why you are going to do it to the patient. Encourage the patient to observe or participate, if possible.	
____	____	____	5. Assemble equipment on the overbed table within reach.	
____	____	____	6. Assist the patient to a comfortable sitting or lying position in bed or a standing or sitting position in the bathroom. If the patient is in bed, adjust the bed to a comfortable working height, usually elbow height of the caregiver. Place a waterproof pad under the patient at the stoma site.	
			Emptying the Appliance	
____	____	____	7. Put on gloves. Hold the end of the appliance over a bedpan, toilet, or measuring device. Remove the end cap from the spout. Open the spout and empty the contents into the bedpan, toilet, or measuring device.	
____	____	____	8. Close the spout. Wipe the spout with toilet tissue. Replace the cap.	
____	____	____	9. Remove equipment. Remove gloves. Assist the patient to a comfortable position.	
____	____	____	10. If appliance is not to be changed, place the bed in the lowest position. Remove additional PPE, if used. Perform hand hygiene.	
			Changing the Appliance	
____	____	____	11. Place a disposable waterproof pad on the overbed table or other work area. Set up the washbasin with warm water and the rest of the supplies. Place a trash bag within reach.	
____	____	____	12. Put on clean gloves. Place waterproof pad under the patient at the stoma site. Empty the appliance if necessary as described in steps 6–8.	

SKILL 36-9

Emptying and Changing a Stoma Appliance
on an Ileal Conduit (Continued)

Excellent	Satisfactory	Needs Practice		Comments
___	___	___	13. Gently remove the appliance, starting at the top and keeping the abdominal skin taut. Remove the appliance faceplate from the skin by pushing the skin from the appliance rather than pulling the appliance from the skin. Apply a silicone-based adhesive remover by spraying or wiping with the remover wipe as needed.	
___	___	___	14. Place the appliance in the trash bag, if disposable. If reusable, set aside to wash in lukewarm soap and water and allow to air dry after the new appliance is in place.	
___	___	___	15. Clean the skin around the stoma with mild skin cleanser and water or a cleansing agent and a washcloth. Remove all old adhesive from the skin; additional adhesive remover may be used. Do not apply lotion to the peristomal area.	
___	___	___	16. Gently pat the area dry. *Make sure the skin around the stoma is thoroughly dry.* Assess the stoma and condition of the surrounding skin.	
___	___	___	17. Place one or two gauze squares over the stoma opening.	
___	___	___	18. Apply skin protectant to a 2-inch (5-cm) radius around the stoma, and allow it to dry completely, which takes about 30 seconds.	
___	___	___	19. Lift the gauze squares for a moment and measure the stoma opening, using the measurement guide. Replace the gauze. Trace the same size opening on the back center of the appliance. Cut the opening 1/8-inch larger than the stoma size. Use a finger to gently smooth the wafer edges after cutting. Check that the spout is closed and the end cap is in place.	
___	___	___	20. Remove the paper backing from the appliance faceplate. Quickly remove the gauze squares and discard appropriately; ease the appliance over the stoma. Gently press onto the skin while smoothing over the surface. Apply gentle, even pressure to the appliance for approximately 30 seconds.	
___	___	___	21. Secure the optional belt to the appliance and around the patient.	
___	___	___	22. Remove gloves. Assist the patient to a comfortable position. Cover the patient with bed linens. Place the bed in the lowest position.	
___	___	___	23. Put on clean gloves. Remove or discard any remaining equipment and assess the patient's response to the procedure.	
___	___	___	24. Remove gloves and additional PPE, if used. Perform hand hygiene.	

Skill Checklists for Fundamentals of Nursing:
The Art and Science of Person-Centered Nursing Care, 8th edition

Name _____   Date _____

Unit _____   Position _____

Instructor/Evaluator: _____   Position _____

SKILL 36-10

Caring for a Hemodialysis Access
(Arteriovenous Fistula or Graft)

Goal: The graft or fistula remains patent; the patient verbalizes appropriate care measures and observations to be made, and demonstrates care measures.

Excellent	Satisfactory	Needs Practice		Comments
___	___	___	1. Perform hand hygiene and put on PPE, if indicated.	
___	___	___	2. Identify the patient.	
___	___	___	3. Close the curtains around the bed and close the door to the room, if possible. Explain what you are going to do, and why you are going to do it, to the patient.	
___	___	___	4. Question the patient about the presence of muscle weakness and cramping; changes in temperature; sensations, such as numbness, tingling, burning, itchiness; and pain.	
___	___	___	5. Inspect the area over the access site for continuity of skin color. Inspect for any redness, warmth, tenderness, edema, rash, blemishes, bleeding, tremors, and twitches. Inspect the muscle strength and the patient's ability to perform range of motion in the extremity/body part with the hemodialysis access.	
___	___	___	6. Palpate over the access site, feeling for a thrill or vibration. Palpate pulses above and below the site. Palpate the continuity of the skin temperature along and around the extremity. Check capillary refill in the fingers or toes of the extremity with the fistula or graft.	
___	___	___	7. Auscultate over the access site with the bell of the stethoscope, listening for a bruit or vibration.	
___	___	___	8. Ensure that a sign is placed over the head of the bed informing the health care team which arm is affected. ***Do not measure blood pressure, perform a venipuncture, or start an IV on the access arm.***	
___	___	___	9. Instruct the patient not to sleep with the arm with the access site under the head or body.	
___	___	___	10. Instruct the patient not to lift heavy objects with, or put pressure on, the arm with the access site. Advise the patient not to carry heavy bags (including purses) on the shoulder of that arm.	
___	___	___	11. Remove PPE, if used. Perform hand hygiene.	

Skill Checklists for Fundamentals of Nursing:
The Art and Science of Person-Centered Nursing Care, 8th edition

Name _____   Date _____

Unit _____   Position _____

Instructor/Evaluator: _____   Position _____

SKILL 36-11

Caring for a Peritoneal Dialysis Catheter

Goal: The peritoneal dialysis catheter dressing change is completed using aseptic technique without trauma to the site or patient; the site is clean, dry, and intact, without evidence of inflammation or infection.

Excellent	Satisfactory	Needs Practice		Comments
____	____	____	1. Review the patient's medical record for orders related to catheter site care. Gather equipment.	
____	____	____	2. Perform hand hygiene and put on PPE, if indicated.	
____	____	____	3. Identify the patient.	
____	____	____	4. Close the curtains around the bed and close the door to the room, if possible. Explain what you are going to do and why you are going to do it to the patient. Encourage the patient to observe or participate if possible.	
____	____	____	5. Assemble equipment on the overbed table within reach.	
____	____	____	6. Adjust bed to comfortable working height, usually elbow height of the caregiver. Assist the patient to a supine position. Expose the abdomen, draping the patient's chest with the bath blanket, exposing only the catheter site.	
____	____	____	7. Put on unsterile gloves. Put on one of the facemasks; have the patient put on the other mask.	
____	____	____	8. Gently remove old dressing, noting odor, amount, and color of drainage, leakage, and condition of the skin around the catheter. Discard the dressing in an appropriate container.	
____	____	____	9. Remove gloves and discard. Set up a sterile field. Open packages. Using aseptic technique, place two sterile gauze squares in a basin with an antimicrobial agent. Leave two sterile gauze squares opened on the sterile field. Alternately (based on facility's policy), place sterile antimicrobial swabs on the sterile field. Place a sterile applicator on the field. Squeeze a small amount of the topical antibiotic on one of the gauze squares on the sterile field.	
____	____	____	10. Put on sterile gloves. Pick up the dialysis catheter with your nondominant hand. *With the antimicrobial-soaked gauze/swab, cleanse the skin around the exit site using a circular motion, starting at the exit site and then slowly going outward 3 to 4 inches. Gently remove crusted scabs, if necessary.*	

SKILL 36-11
Caring for a Peritoneal Dialysis Catheter *(Continued)*

Excellent	Satisfactory	Needs Practice		Comments
——	——	——	11. *Continue to hold the catheter with your nondominant hand. After the skin has dried, clean the catheter with an antimicrobial-soaked gauze, beginning at the exit site, going around the catheter, and then moving up to the end of the catheter. Gently remove crusted secretions on the tube, if necessary.*	
——	——	——	12. Using the sterile applicator, apply the topical antibiotic to the catheter exit site, if prescribed.	
——	——	——	13. Place a sterile drain sponge around the exit site. Then place a 4 × 4 gauze over the exit site. Cover with transparent, occlusive dressing. Remove masks.	
——	——	——	14. Label the dressing with date, time of change, and your initials.	
——	——	——	15. Coil the exposed length of tubing and secure to the dressing or the patient's abdomen with tape.	
——	——	——	16. Assist the patient to a comfortable position. Cover the patient with bed linens. Place the bed in the lowest position.	
——	——	——	17. Put on clean gloves. Remove or discard equipment and assess the patient's response to the procedure.	
——	——	——	18. Remove gloves and additional PPE, if used. Perform hand hygiene.	

Skill Checklists for Fundamentals of Nursing:
The Art and Science of Person-Centered Nursing Care, 8th edition

Name _____   Date _____

Unit _____   Position _____

Instructor/Evaluator: _____   Position _____

SKILL 37-1

Administering a Large-Volume Cleansing Enema

Goal: The patient expels feces and is free from injury with minimal discomfort.

Columns: Excellent | Satisfactory | Needs Practice | | Comments

Excellent	Satisfactory	Needs Practice		Comments
___	___	___	1. Verify the order for the enema. Gather equipment.	
___	___	___	2. Perform hand hygiene and put on PPE, if indicated.	
___	___	___	3. Identify the patient.	
___	___	___	4. Explain the procedure to the patient and provide the rationale as to why the tube is needed. Discuss the associated discomforts that may be experienced and possible interventions that may allay this discomfort. Answer any questions as needed.	
___	___	___	5. Assemble equipment on the overbed table within reach.	
___	___	___	6. Close the curtains around the bed and close the door to the room, if possible. Discuss where the patient will defecate. Have a bedpan, commode, or nearby bathroom ready for use.	
___	___	___	7. Warm the enema solution in the amount ordered, and check the temperature with a bath thermometer, if available. If a bath thermometer is not available, warm to room temperature or slightly higher, and test on the inner wrist. If tap water is used, adjust temperature as it flows from the faucet.	
___	___	___	8. Add the enema solution to the container. Release the clamp and allow the fluid to progress through the tube before reclamping.	
___	___	___	9. Adjust the bed to a comfortable working height, usually elbow height of the caregiver. Position the patient on the left side (Sims position), as dictated by patient comfort and condition. Fold top linen back just enough to allow access to the patient's rectal area. Drape the patient with the bath blanket as necessary to maintain privacy and warmth. Place a waterproof pad under the patient's hip.	
___	___	___	10. Put on gloves.	
___	___	___	11. Elevate solution so that it is no higher than 18 inches (45 cm) above level of anus. Plan to give the solution slowly over a period of 5 to 10 minutes. Hang the container on an IV pole or hold it at the proper height.	

Excellent	Satisfactory	Needs Practice	SKILL 37-1 **Administering a Large-Volume Cleansing Enema** *(Continued)*	
				Comments
——	——	——	12. Generously lubricate the end of the rectal tube 2 to 3 inches (5–7 cm). A disposable enema set may have a prelubricated rectal tube.	
——	——	——	13. Lift the buttock to expose the anus. Ask the patient to take several deep breaths. Slowly and gently insert the enema tube 3 to 4 inches (7–10 cm) for an adult. Direct it at an angle pointing toward the umbilicus, not the bladder.	
——	——	——	14. If resistance is met while inserting the tube, permit a small amount of solution to enter, withdraw tube slightly, and then continue to insert it. *Do not force entry of the tube.* Ask the patient to take several deep breaths.	
——	——	——	15. Introduce solution slowly over a period of 5 to 10 minutes. Hold the tubing all the time that the solution is being instilled. Assess for dizziness, lightheadedness, nausea, diaphoresis, and clammy skin during administration. *If the patient experiences any of these symptoms, stop the procedure immediately, monitor the patient's heart rate and blood pressure, and notify the primary care provider.*	
——	——	——	16. Clamp the tubing or lower container if the patient has the urge to defecate or cramping occurs. Instruct the patient to take small, fast breaths or to pant.	
——	——	——	17. After solution has been given, clamp the tubing and remove the tube. Have a paper towel ready to receive the tube as it is withdrawn.	
——	——	——	18. Return the patient to a comfortable position. Encourage the patient to hold the solution until the urge to defecate is strong, usually in about 5 to 15 minutes. Make sure the linens under the patient are dry. Remove your gloves and ensure that the patient is covered.	
——	——	——	19. Raise the side rail. Lower the bed height and adjust the head of the bed to a comfortable position.	
——	——	——	20. Remove additional PPE, if used. Perform hand hygiene.	
——	——	——	21. When the patient has a strong urge to defecate, place the patient in a sitting position on a bedpan or assist to the commode or bathroom. Offer toilet tissues, if not in the patient's reach. Stay with the patient or have the call bell readily accessible.	

SKILL 37-1

Administering a Large-Volume Cleansing Enema *(Continued)*

Excellent	Satisfactory	Needs Practice		Comments
——	——	——	22. Remind the patient not to flush the commode before you inspect the results of the enema.	
——	——	——	23. Put on gloves and assist the patient, if necessary, with cleaning of the anal area. Offer washcloths, skin cleanser, and water for handwashing. Remove gloves.	
——	——	——	24. Leave the patient clean and comfortable. Care for equipment properly.	
——	——	——	25. Perform hand hygiene.	

Name _____ Date _____

Unit _____ Position _____

Instructor/Evaluator: _____ Position _____

SKILL 37-2

Irrigating a Nasogastric Tube Connected to Suction

Goal: The tube maintains patency with irrigation and patient remains free from injury.

Excellent	Satisfactory	Needs Practice		Comments
___	___	___	1. Gather equipment. Verify the medical order or facility policy and procedure regarding frequency of irrigation, solution type, and amount of irrigant. Check expiration dates on irrigating solution and irrigation set.	
___	___	___	2. Perform hand hygiene and put on PPE, if indicated.	
___	___	___	3. Identify the patient.	
___	___	___	4. Explain the procedure to the patient and why this intervention is needed. Answer any questions as needed. Perform key abdominal assessments.	
___	___	___	5. Assemble equipment on the overbed table within reach.	
___	___	___	6. Pull the patient's bedside curtain. Raise the bed to a comfortable working position, usually elbow height of the caregiver. Assist the patient to a 30- to 45-degree position, unless this is contraindicated. Pour the irrigating solution into a container.	
___	___	___	7. Put on gloves. Place a waterproof pad on the patient's chest, under the connection of the nasogastric tube and suction tubing. *Check placement of the NG tube.*	
___	___	___	8. Draw up 30 mL of irrigation solution (or the amount indicated in the order or policy) into a syringe.	
___	___	___	9. Clamp the nasogastric tube near the connection site. Disconnect the tube from the suction apparatus and lay on disposable pad or towel, or hold both tubes upright in your nondominant hand.	
___	___	___	10. Place the tip of the syringe in the tube. *If a Salem sump or double-lumen tube is used, make sure that the syringe tip is placed in the drainage port and not in the blue air vent.* Hold the syringe upright and gently insert the irrigant, or allow the solution to flow in by gravity if facility policy or medical order indicates. *Do not force the solution into the tube.*	

Irrigating a Nasogastric Tube
Connected to Suction *(Continued)*

Excellent	Satisfactory	Needs Practice		Comments
—	—	—	11. *If unable to irrigate the tube, reposition the patient and attempt irrigation again. Inject 10 to 20 mL of air and aspirate again. If repeated attempts to irrigate the tube fail, consult with the primary care provider or follow facility policy.*	
—	—	—	12. After irrigant has been instilled, hold the end of the NG tube over an irrigation tray or emesis basin. Observe for return flow of NG drainage into an available container. Alternately, you may reconnect the NG tube to suction and observe the return drainage as it drains into the suction container.	
—	—	—	13. If not already done, reconnect the drainage port to the suction, if ordered.	
—	—	—	14. Inject air into the blue air vent after irrigation is complete. Position the blue air vent above the patient's stomach.	
—	—	—	15. Remove gloves. Lower the bed and raise the side rails, as necessary. Assist the patient to a position of comfort. Perform hand hygiene.	
—	—	—	16. Put on gloves. Measure the returned solution, if collected outside of the suction apparatus. Rinse equipment if it will be reused. Label with the date, patient's name, room number, and purpose (for NG tube/irrigation).	
—	—	—	17. Remove gloves and additional PPE, if used. Perform hand hygiene.	

Skill Checklists for Fundamentals of Nursing:
The Art and Science of Person-Centered Nursing Care, 8th edition

Name _____   Date _____

Unit _____   Position _____

Instructor/Evaluator: _____   Position _____

SKILL 37-3

Changing and Emptying an Ostomy Appliance

Excellent	Satisfactory	Needs Practice	**Goal:** The stoma appliance is applied correctly to the skin to allow stool to drain freely.	Comments
____	____	____	1. Gather equipment.	
____	____	____	2. Perform hand hygiene and put on PPE, if indicated.	
____	____	____	3. Identify the patient.	
____	____	____	4. Close curtains around the bed and close the door to the room, if possible. Explain what you are going to do and why you are going to do it to the patient. Encourage the patient to observe or participate, if possible.	
____	____	____	5. Assemble equipment on the overbed table within reach.	
____	____	____	6. Assist the patient to a comfortable sitting or lying position in bed or a standing or sitting position in the bathroom. If the patient is in bed, adjust the bed to a comfortable working height, usually elbow height of the caregiver. Place a waterproof pad under the patient at the stoma site.	
			Emptying an Appliance	
____	____	____	7. Put on disposable gloves. Remove the clamp and fold the end of the appliance or pouch upward like a cuff.	
____	____	____	8. Empty contents into a bedpan, toilet, or measuring device.	
____	____	____	9. Wipe the lower 2 inches of the appliance or pouch with toilet tissue or paper towel.	
____	____	____	10. Uncuff the edge of the appliance or pouch and apply the clip or clamp, or secure the Velcro closure. Ensure that the curve of the clamp follows the curve of the patient's body. Remove gloves. Assist the patient to a comfortable position.	
____	____	____	11. If the appliance is not to be changed, remove additional PPE, if used. Perform hand hygiene.	
			Changing an Appliance	
____	____	____	12. Place a disposable pad on the work surface. Set up the washbasin with warm water and the rest of the supplies. Place a trash bag within reach.	
____	____	____	13. Put on clean gloves. Place a waterproof pad under the patient at the stoma site. Empty the appliance as described previously.	

Changing and Emptying an Ostomy Appliance *(Continued)*

Excellent	Satisfactory	Needs Practice		Comments

___	___	___	14. Start at the top of the appliance and keep the abdominal skin taut. Gently remove the pouch faceplate from the skin by pushing the skin from the appliance rather than pulling the appliance from the skin. Apply a silicone-based adhesive remover by spraying or wiping with the remover wipe.	
___	___	___	15. Place the appliance in the trash bag, if disposable. If reusable, set aside to wash in lukewarm soap and water, and allow to air dry after the new appliance is in place.	
___	___	___	16. Use toilet tissue to remove any excess stool from the stoma. Cover the stoma with a gauze pad. Clean the skin around the stoma with skin cleanser and water or a cleansing agent and a washcloth. Remove all old adhesive from the skin; use an adhesive remover, as necessary. Do not apply lotion to the peristomal area.	
___	___	___	17. Gently pat area dry. *Make sure that the skin around the stoma is thoroughly dry.* Assess the stoma and the condition of the surrounding skin.	
___	___	___	18. Apply skin protectant to a 2-inch (5-cm) radius around the stoma, and allow it to dry completely, which takes about 30 seconds.	
___	___	___	19. Lift the gauze squares for a moment and measure the stoma opening, using the measurement guide. Replace the gauze. Trace the same-size opening on the back center of the appliance. Cut the opening 1/8 inch larger than the stoma size. Use a finger to gently smooth the wafer edges after cutting.	
___	___	___	20. Remove the paper backing from the appliance faceplate. Quickly remove the gauze squares and case the appliance over the stoma. Gently press onto the skin while smoothing over the surface. Apply gentle, even pressure to the appliance for approximately 30 seconds.	
___	___	___	21. Close the bottom of the appliance or pouch by folding the end upward and using the clamp or clip that comes with the product, or secure the Velcro closure. Ensure that the curve of the clamp follows the curve of the patient's body.	
___	___	___	22. Remove gloves. Assist the patient to a comfortable position. Cover the patient with bed linens. Place the bed in the lowest position.	
___	___	___	23. Put on clean gloves. Remove or discard equipment and assess the patient's response to the procedure.	
___	___	___	24. Remove gloves and additional PPE, if used. Perform hand hygiene.	

Skill Checklists for Fundamentals of Nursing:
The Art and Science of Person-Centered Nursing Care, 8th edition

Name _____   Date _____

Unit _____   Position _____

Instructor/Evaluator: _____   Position _____

Excellent	Satisfactory	Needs Practice	SKILL 38-1 **Using a Pulse Oximeter**	Comments
			Goal: The patient exhibits arterial blood oxygen saturation within acceptable parameters, or greater than 95%.	
___	___	___	1. Review the health record for any health problems that would affect the patient's oxygenation status.	
___	___	___	2. Bring necessary equipment to the bedside stand or overbed table.	
___	___	___	3. Perform hand hygiene and put on PPE, if indicated.	
___	___	___	4. Identify the patient.	
___	___	___	5. Close the curtains around the bed and close the door to the room, if possible. Explain what you are going to do and why you are going to do it to the patient.	
___	___	___	6. Select an adequate site for application of the sensor.	
___	___	___	a. Use the patient's index, middle, or ring finger.	
___	___	___	b. Check the proximal pulse and capillary refill at the pulse closest to the site.	
___	___	___	c. If circulation at the site is inadequate, consider using the earlobe, forehead, or bridge of the nose. Use the appropriate oximetry sensor for the chosen site.	
___	___	___	d. Use a toe only if lower extremity circulation is not compromised.	
___	___	___	7. Select proper equipment:	
___	___	___	a. If one finger is too large for the probe, use a smaller finger.	
___	___	___	b. Use probes appropriate for the patient's age and size. Use a pediatric probe for a small adult, if necessary.	
___	___	___	c. Check if the patient is allergic to adhesive. A nonadhesive finger clip or reflectance sensor is available.	
___	___	___	8. Prepare the monitoring site. Cleanse the selected area with an alcohol wipe or disposable cleansing cloth. Allow the area to dry. If necessary, remove nail polish and artificial nails after checking the pulse oximeter's manufacturer instructions.	
___	___	___	9. *Apply probe securely to skin. Make sure that the light-emitting sensor and the light-receiving sensor are aligned opposite each other (not necessary to check if placed on the forehead or bridge of the nose).*	

SKILL 38-1

Using a Pulse Oximeter *(Continued)*

Excellent	Satisfactory	Needs Practice		Comments
⎯⎯	⎯⎯	⎯⎯	10. Connect the sensor probe to the pulse oximeter, turn the oximeter on, and check operation of the equipment (audible beep, fluctuation of bar of light or waveform on face of oximeter).	
⎯⎯	⎯⎯	⎯⎯	11. Set the alarms on the pulse oximeter. Check the manufacturer's alarm limits for high and low pulse rate settings.	
⎯⎯	⎯⎯	⎯⎯	12. Check oxygen saturation at regular intervals, as ordered the by primary care provider, nursing assessment, and signaled by alarms. Monitor hemoglobin level.	
⎯⎯	⎯⎯	⎯⎯	13. Remove the sensor on a regular basis and check for skin irritation or signs of pressure (every 2 hours for a spring-tension sensor or every 4 hours for an adhesive finger or toe sensor).	
⎯⎯	⎯⎯	⎯⎯	14. Clean nondisposable sensors according to the manufacturer's directions. Remove PPE, if used. Perform hand hygiene.	

Skill Checklists for Fundamentals of Nursing:
The Art and Science of Person-Centered Nursing Care, 8th edition

Name _____ Date _____

Unit _____ Position _____

Instructor/Evaluator: _____ Position _____

Excellent	Satisfactory	Needs Practice	SKILL 38-2 **Suctioning the Oropharyngeal and Nasopharyngeal Airways**	
			Goal: The patient exhibits improved breath sounds and a clear, patent airway.	**Comments**
___	___	___	1. Bring necessary equipment to the bedside stand or overbed table.	
___	___	___	2. Perform hand hygiene and put on PPE, if indicated.	
___	___	___	3. Identify the patient.	
___	___	___	4. Close the curtains around the bed and close the door to the room, if possible.	
			5. Determine the need for suctioning. Verify the suction order in the patient's medical record, if necessary. *Assess for pain or the potential to cause pain. Administer pain medication, as prescribed, before suctioning.*	
			6. Explain what you are going to do and the reason for suctioning to the patient, even if the patient does not appear to be alert. Reassure the patient that you will interrupt procedure if the patient indicates respiratory difficulty.	
___	___	___	7. Adjust the bed to a comfortable working height, usually elbow height of the caregiver. Lower the side rail closest to you. *If the patient is conscious, place him or her in a semi-Fowler's position. If patient is unconscious, place him or her in the lateral position, facing you.* Move the bedside table close to your work area and raise it to waist height.	
___			8. Place a towel or waterproof pad across the patient's chest.	
___	___	___	9. *Adjust suction to the appropriate pressure.*	
			For a wall unit for an adult: 100–150 mm Hg; neonates: 60–80 mm Hg; infants: 80–125 mm Hg; children: 80–125 mm Hg; adolescents: 80–150 mm Hg (Hess, 2012).	
___	___	___	For a portable unit for an adult: 10–15 cm Hg; neonates: 6–8 cm Hg; infants: 8–10 cm Hg; children: 8–10 cm Hg; adolescents: 8–15 cm Hg.	
___	___	___	*Put on a disposable, clean glove and occlude the end of the connecting tubing to check suction pressure.* Place the connecting tubing in a convenient location.	

Excellent	Satisfactory	Needs Practice	

Comments

——	——	——	10. Open a sterile suction package using aseptic technique. The open wrapper or container becomes a sterile field to hold other supplies. Carefully remove the sterile container, touching only the outside surface. Set it up on the work surface and pour sterile saline into it.
——	——	——	11. Place a small amount of water-soluble lubricant on the sterile field, taking care to avoid touching the sterile field with the lubricant package.
——	——	——	12. Increase the patient's supplemental oxygen level or apply supplemental oxygen per facility policy or primary care provider order.
——	——	——	13. Put on a face shield or goggles and mask. Put on sterile gloves. *The dominant hand will manipulate the catheter and must remain sterile. The nondominant hand is considered clean rather than sterile and will control the suction valve (Y-port) on the catheter.* In the home setting and other community-based settings, maintenance of sterility is not necessary.
——	——	——	14. With your dominant gloved hand, pick up the sterile catheter. Pick up the connecting tubing with your nondominant hand and connect the tubing and suction catheter.
——	——	——	15. Moisten the catheter by dipping it into the container of sterile saline. Occlude the Y-tube to check suction.
——	——	——	16. Encourage the patient to take several deep breaths.
——	——	——	17. Apply lubricant to the first 2 to 3 inches of the catheter, using the lubricant that was placed on the sterile field.
——	——	——	18. Remove the oxygen delivery device, if appropriate. Do not apply suction as the catheter is inserted. Hold the catheter between your thumb and forefinger.
			19. Insert the catheter:
——	——	——	a. **For nasopharyngeal suctioning,** gently insert the catheter through the naris and along the floor of the nostril toward the trachea. Roll the catheter between your fingers to help advance it. Advance the catheter approximately 5 to 6 inches to reach the pharynx.
——	——	——	b. **For oropharyngeal suctioning,** insert the catheter through the mouth, along the side of the mouth toward the trachea. Advance the catheter 3″ to 4″ to reach the pharynx.

SKILL 38-2

Suctioning the Oropharyngeal and Nasopharyngeal Airways *(Continued)*

Excellent	Satisfactory	Needs Practice		Comments

——	——	——	20. *Apply suction by intermittently occluding the Y-port on the catheter with the thumb of your nondominant hand and gently rotating the catheter as it is being withdrawn. Do not suction for more than 10 to 15 seconds at a time.*	
——	——	——	21. Replace the oxygen delivery device using your nondominant hand, if appropriate, and have the patient take several deep breaths.	
——	——	——	22. Flush the catheter with saline. Assess effectiveness of suctioning and repeat, as needed, according to the patient's tolerance. Wrap the suction catheter around your dominant hand between attempts.	
——	——	——	23. *Allow at least a 30-second to 1-minute interval if additional suctioning is needed. No more than three suction passes should be made per suctioning episode. Alternate the nares, unless contraindicated, if repeated suctioning is required.* Do not force the catheter through the nares. Encourage the patient to cough and deep breathe between suctioning. *Suction the oropharynx after suctioning the nasopharynx.*	
——	——	——	24. When suctioning is completed, remove gloves from your dominant hand over the coiled catheter, pulling them off inside out. Remove the glove from your nondominant hand and dispose of gloves, catheter, and container with solution in the appropriate receptacle. Assist the patient to a comfortable position. Raise the bed rail and place the bed in the lowest position.	
——	——	——	25. Turn off suction. Remove the supplemental oxygen placed for suctioning, if appropriate. Remove the face shield or goggles and mask. Perform hand hygiene.	
——	——	——	26. Offer oral hygiene after suctioning.	
——	——	——	27. Reassess the patient's respiratory status, including respiratory rate, effort, oxygen saturation, and lung sounds.	
——	——	——	28. Remove additional PPE, if used. Perform hand hygiene.	

Skill Checklists for Fundamentals of Nursing:
The Art and Science of Person-Centered Nursing Care, 8th edition

Name _____   Date _____

Unit _____   Position _____

Instructor/Evaluator: _____   Position _____

Excellent	Satisfactory	Needs Practice	SKILL 38-3 **Administering Oxygen by Nasal Cannula**	Comments
			Goal: The patient exhibits an oxygen saturation level within acceptable parameters.	
――	――	――	1. Bring necessary equipment to the bedside stand or overbed table.	
――	――	――	2. Perform hand hygiene and put on PPE, if indicated.	
――	――	――	3. Identify the patient.	
――	――	――	4. Close the curtains around the bed and close the door to the room, if possible.	
――	――	――	5. Explain what you are going to do and the reason for doing it to the patient. Review safety precautions necessary when oxygen is in use.	
――	――	――	6. Connect nasal cannula to oxygen setup with humidification, if humidification is in use. Adjust flow rate as ordered. Check that oxygen is flowing out of the prongs.	
――	――	――	7. Place the prongs in the patient's nostrils. Place the tubing over and behind each ear with the adjuster comfortably under the chin. Alternately, the tubing may be placed around the patient's head, with the adjuster at the back or base of the head. Place gauze pads at the ear beneath the tubing, as necessary.	
――	――	――	8. Adjust the fit of the cannula, as necessary. Tubing should be snug but not tight against the skin.	
――	――	――	9. *Encourage patients to breathe through the nose, with the mouth closed.*	
――	――	――	10. Reassess the patient's respiratory status, including respiratory rate, effort, and lung sounds. Note any signs of respiratory distress, such as tachypnea, nasal flaring, use of accessory muscles, or dyspnea.	
――	――	――	11. Remove PPE, if used. Perform hand hygiene.	
――	――	――	12. Put on clean gloves. Remove and clean the cannula and assess nares at least every 8 hours, or according to agency recommendations. Check nares for evidence of irritation or bleeding.	

Skill Checklists for Fundamentals of Nursing:
The Art and Science of Person-Centered Nursing Care, 8th edition

Name _____ Date _____

Unit _____ Position _____

Instructor/Evaluator: _____ Position _____

Excellent	Satisfactory	Needs Practice	SKILL 38-4 **Administering Oxygen by Mask** **Goal:** The patient exhibits an oxygen saturation level within acceptable parameters.	Comments
——	——	——	1. Bring necessary equipment to the bedside stand or overbed table.	
——	——	——	2. Perform hand hygiene and put on PPE, if indicated.	
——	——	——	3. Identify the patient.	
——	——	——	4. Close the curtains around the bed and close the door to the room, if possible.	
——	——	——	5. Explain what you are going to do and the reason for doing it to the patient. Review safety precautions necessary when oxygen is in use.	
——	——	——	6. Attach the face mask to the oxygen source (with humidification, if appropriate, for the specific mask). Start the flow of oxygen at the specified rate. For a mask with a reservoir, be sure to allow oxygen to fill the bag before proceeding to the next step.	
——	——	——	7. Position the face mask over the patient's nose and mouth. Adjust the elastic strap so that the mask fits snugly but comfortably on the face. Adjust the flow rate to the prescribed rate.	
——	——	——	8. If the patient reports irritation or you note redness, use gauze pads under the elastic strap at pressure points to reduce irritation to ears and scalp.	
——	——	——	9. Reassess the patient's respiratory status, including respiratory rate, effort, and lung sounds. Note any signs of respiratory distress, such as tachypnea, nasal flaring, use of accessory muscles, or dyspnea.	
——	——	——	10. Remove PPE, if used. Perform hand hygiene.	
——	——	——	11. *Remove the mask and dry the skin every 2 to 3 hours if the oxygen is running continuously. Do not use powder around the mask.*	

Skill Checklists for Fundamentals of Nursing:
The Art and Science of Person-Centered Nursing Care, 8th edition

Name _____   Date _____

Unit _____   Position _____

Instructor/Evaluator: _____   Position _____

SKILL 38-5

Providing Care of a Tracheostomy Tube

Goal: The patient exhibits a tracheostomy tube and site free from drainage, secretions, and skin irritation or breakdown.

Excellent	Satisfactory	Needs Practice		Comments
——	——	——	1. Bring necessary equipment to the bedside stand or overbed table.	
——	——	——	2. Perform hand hygiene and put on PPE, if indicated.	
——	——	——	3. Identify the patient.	
——	——	——	4. Close the curtains around the bed and close the door to the room, if possible.	
——	——	——	5. Determine the need for tracheostomy care. *Assess the patient's pain and administer pain medication, if indicated.*	
——	——	——	6. Explain what you are going to do and the reason for doing it to the patient, even if the patient does not appear to be alert. Reassure the patient that you will interrupt procedure if he or she indicates respiratory difficulty.	
——	——	——	7. Adjust the bed to a comfortable working position, usually elbow height of the caregiver. Lower the side rail closest to you. *If the patient is conscious, place him or her in a semi-Fowler's position. If patient is unconscious, place him or her in the lateral position, facing you.* Move the overbed table close to your work area and raise it to waist height. Place a trash receptacle within easy reach of the work area.	
——	——	——	8. Put on a face shield or goggles and mask. Suction the tracheostomy, if necessary. If the tracheostomy has just been suctioned, remove the soiled site dressing and discard before removal of gloves used to perform suctioning.	
			Cleaning the Tracheostomy: Disposable Inner Cannula	
——	——	——	9. Carefully open the package with the new disposable inner cannula, taking care not to contaminate the cannula or the inside of the package. Carefully open the package with the sterile cotton-tipped applicators, taking care not to contaminate them. Open a sterile cup or basin and fill 0.5 inch deep with saline. Open the plastic disposable bag and place within reach on the work surface.	
——	——	——	10. Put on disposable gloves.	

SKILL 38-5

Providing Care of a Tracheostomy Tube *(Continued)*

Excellent	Satisfactory	Needs Practice		Comments

—— —— ——			11. Remove the oxygen source if one is present. Stabilize the outer cannula and faceplate of the tracheostomy with your nondominant hand. Grasp the locking mechanism of the inner cannula with your dominant hand. Press the tabs and release the lock. Gently remove the inner cannula and place in a disposal bag. If not already removed, remove the site dressing and dispose of it in the trash.
—— —— ——			12. Discard gloves and put on sterile gloves. Pick up the new inner cannula with your dominant hand, stabilize the face-plate with your nondominant hand, and gently insert the new inner cannula into the outer cannula. Press the tabs to allow the lock to grab the outer cannula. Reapply the oxygen source, if needed.

Applying Clean Dressing and Holder

—— —— ——			13. Remove the oxygen source, if necessary. Dip a cotton-tipped applicator or gauze sponge in a cup or basin with sterile saline and clean the stoma under the faceplate. Use each applicator or sponge only once, moving from the stoma site outward.
—— —— ——			14. Pat skin gently with a dry 4 × 4 gauze sponge.
—— —— ——			15. Slide a commercially prepared tracheostomy dressing or prefolded non–cotton-filled 4 × 4-inch dressing under the faceplate.
—— —— ——			16. Change the tracheostomy holder:
—— —— ——			a. *Obtain the assistance of a second person to hold the tracheostomy tube in place while the old collar is removed and the new collar is placed.*
—— —— ——			b. Open the package for the new tracheostomy collar.
—— —— ——			c. Both nurses should put on clean gloves.
—— —— ——			d. One nurse holds the faceplate while the other pulls up the Velcro tabs. Gently remove the collar.
—— —— ——			e. The first nurse continues to hold the tracheostomy faceplate.
—— —— ——			f. The other nurse places the collar around the patient's neck and inserts first one tab, then the other, into the openings on the faceplate and secures the Velcro tabs on the tracheostomy holder.
—— —— ——			g. Check the fit of the tracheostomy collar. You should be able to fit one finger between the neck and the collar. Check to make sure that the patient can flex the neck comfortably. Reapply the oxygen source, if necessary.

Providing Care of a Tracheostomy Tube *(Continued)*

Excellent	Satisfactory	Needs Practice		Comments
___	___	___	17. Remove gloves. Remove the face shield or goggles and mask. Assist the patient to a comfortable position. Raise the bed rail and place the bed in the lowest position.	
___	___	___	18. Reassess patient's respiratory status, including respiratory rate, effort, oxygen saturation, and lung sounds.	
___	___	___	19. Remove additional PPE, if used. Perform hand hygiene.	

Skill Checklists for Fundamentals of Nursing:
The Art and Science of Person-Centered Nursing Care, 8th edition

Name _____ Date _____

Unit _____ Position _____

Instructor/Evaluator: _____ Position _____

SKILL 38-6

Suctioning a Tracheostomy: Open System

Excellent	Satisfactory	Needs Practice	**Goal:** The patient exhibits improved breath sounds and a clear, patent airway.	Comments
——	——	——	1. Bring necessary equipment to the bedside stand or overbed table.	
——	——	——	2. Perform hand hygiene and put on PPE, if indicated.	
——	——	——	3. Identify the patient.	
——	——	——	4. Close curtains around the bed and close the door to the room, if possible.	
——	——	——	5. Determine the need for suctioning. Verify the suction order in the patient's medical record. *Assess for pain or the potential to cause pain. Administer pain medication, as prescribed, before suctioning.*	
——	——	——	6. Explain to the patient what you are going to do and the reason for doing it, even if the patient does not appear to be alert. Reassure the patient that you will interrupt the procedure if the patient indicates respiratory difficulty.	
——	——	——	7. Adjust the bed to a comfortable working position, usually elbow height of the caregiver. Lower the side rail closest to you. *If the patient is conscious, place the patient in a semi-Fowler's position. If unconscious, place him or her in the lateral position, facing you.* Move the overbed table close to your work area and raise it to waist height.	
——	——	——	8. Place a towel or waterproof pad across the patient's chest.	
——	——	——	9. Turn the suction to the appropriate pressure.	
——	——	——	For a wall unit for an adult: 100–150 mm Hg; neonates: 60–80 mm Hg; infants: 80–125 mm Hg; children: 80–125 mm Hg; adolescents: 80–150 mm Hg (Hess, 2012).	
——	——	——	For a portable unit for an adult: 10–15 cm Hg; neonates: 6–8 cm Hg; infants: 8–10 cm Hg; children: 8–10 cm Hg; adolescents: 8–15 cm Hg.	
——	——	——	Put on a disposable, clean glove and occlude the end of the connecting tubing to check suction pressure. Place the connecting tubing in a convenient location. If using, place the resuscitation bag connected to the oxygen within convenient reach.	

Suctioning a Tracheostomy: Open System *(Continued)*

Excellent	Satisfactory	Needs Practice		Comments
——	——	——	10. Open a sterile suction package using aseptic technique. The open wrapper or container becomes a sterile field to hold other supplies. Carefully remove the sterile container, touching only the outside surface. Set it up on the work surface and pour sterile saline into it.	
——	——	——	11. Put on a face shield or goggles and mask. Put on sterile gloves. *The dominant hand will manipulate the catheter and must remain sterile. The nondominant hand is considered clean rather than sterile and will control the suction valve (Y-port) on the catheter.*	
——	——	——	12. With your dominant gloved hand, pick up the sterile catheter. Pick up the connecting tubing with your nondominant hand and connect the tubing and suction catheter.	
——	——	——	13. Moisten the catheter by dipping it into the container of sterile saline, unless it is a silicone catheter. Occlude the Y-tube to check the suction.	
——	——	——	14. Using your nondominant hand and a manual resuscitation bag, hyperventilate the patient, delivering three to six breaths or use the sigh mechanism on a mechanical ventilator.	
——	——	——	15. Open the adapter on the mechanical ventilator tubing or remove the oxygen delivery setup with your nondominant hand.	
——	——	——	16. Using your dominant hand, gently and quickly insert the catheter into the trachea. *Advance the catheter to the predetermined length. Do not occlude the Y-port when inserting the catheter.*	
——	——	——	17. Apply suction by intermittently occluding the Y-port on the catheter with the thumb of your nondominant hand, and gently rotate the catheter as it is being withdrawn. *Do not suction for more than 10 to 15 seconds at a time.*	
——	——	——	18. Hyperventilate the patient using your nondominant hand and a manual resuscitation bag, delivering three to six breaths. Replace the oxygen delivery device, if applicable, using your nondominant hand and have the patient take several deep breaths. If the patient is mechanically ventilated, close the adapter on the mechanical ventilator tubing and use the sigh mechanism on a mechanical ventilator.	
——	——	——	19. Flush the catheter with saline. Assess the effectiveness of suctioning and repeat, as needed, according to the patient's tolerance. Wrap the suction catheter around your dominant hand between attempts.	

SKILL 38-6

Suctioning a Tracheostomy: Open System *(Continued)*

Excellent	Satisfactory	Needs Practice		Comments
——	——	——	20. *Allow at least a 30-second to 1-minute interval if additional suctioning is needed. Do not make more than three suction passes per suctioning episode. Encourage the patient to cough and deep breathe between suctioning attempts.* Suction the oropharynx after suctioning the trachea. Do not reinsert in the tracheostomy after suctioning the mouth.	
——	——	——	21. When suctioning is completed, remove the glove from your dominant hand over the coiled catheter, pulling it off inside out. Remove the glove from your nondominant hand and dispose of gloves, catheter, and container with solution in the appropriate receptacle. Assist the patient to a comfortable position. Raise the bed rail and place the bed in the lowest position.	
——	——	——	22. Turn off the suction. Remove the supplemental oxygen placed for suctioning, if appropriate. Remove the face shield or goggles and mask. Perform hand hygiene.	
——	——	——	23. Offer oral hygiene after suctioning.	
——	——	——	24. Reassess the patient's respiratory status, including respiratory rate, effort, oxygen saturation, and lung sounds.	
——	——	——	25. Remove additional PPE, if used. Perform hand hygiene.	

Skill Checklists for Fundamentals of Nursing:
The Art and Science of Person-Centered Nursing Care, 8th edition

Name _____ Date _____

Unit _____ Position _____

Instructor/Evaluator: _____ Position _____

Excellent	Satisfactory	Needs Practice	SKILL 39-1 **Initiating a Peripheral Venous Access IV Infusion**	Comments
			Goal: The access device is inserted on the first attempt, using sterile technique.	
——	——	——	1. Verify the IV solution order on the MAR/CMAR with the medical order. Consider the appropriateness of the prescribed therapy in relation to the patient. Clarify any inconsistencies. Check the patient's chart for allergies. Check for color, leaking, and expiration date. Know techniques for IV insertion, precautions, purpose of the IV administration, and medications if ordered. Gather necessary supplies.	
——	——	——	2. Perform hand hygiene and put on PPE, if indicated.	
——	——	——	3. Identify the patient.	
——	——	——	4. Close the curtains around the bed and close the door to the room, if possible. Explain what you are going to do and why you are going to do it to the patient. Ask the patient about allergies to medications, tape, or skin antiseptics, as appropriate. If considering using a local anesthetic, inquire about allergies for these substances as well.	
——	——	——	5. If using a local anesthetic, explain the rationale and procedure to the patient. Apply the anesthetic to a few potential insertion sites. Allow sufficient time for the anesthetic to take effect.	
			Prepare the IV Solution and Administration Set	
——	——	——	6. Compare the IV container label with the MAR/CMAR. Remove the IV bag from the outer wrapper, if indicated. Check expiration dates. Scan the bar code on the container, if necessary. Compare the patient identification band with the MAR/CMAR. Alternately, label the solution container with the patient's name, solution type, additives, date, and time. Complete a time strip for the infusion and apply to the IV container.	
——	——	——	7. Maintain aseptic technique when opening sterile packages and the IV solution. Remove the administration set from the package. Apply the label to the tubing, reflecting the day/date for next set change, per facility guidelines.	

Initiating a Peripheral Venous Access
IV Infusion *(Continued)*

Excellent	Satisfactory	Needs Practice		Comments

8. Close the roller clamp or slide clamp on the IV administration set. Invert the IV solution container and remove the cap on the entry site, taking care not to touch the exposed entry site. Remove the cap from the spike on the administration set. Using a twisting and pushing motion, insert the administration set spike into the entry site of the IV container. Alternately, follow the manufacturer's directions for insertion.

9. Hang the IV container on the IV pole. Squeeze the drip chamber and fill at least halfway.

10. Open the IV tubing clamp, and allow fluid to move through tubing. Follow additional manufacturer's instructions for specific electronic infusion pump, as indicated. *Allow fluid to flow until all air bubbles have disappeared and the entire length of the tubing is primed (filled) with IV solution.* Close the clamp. Alternately, some brands of tubing may require removal of the cap at the end of the IV tubing to allow fluid to flow. Maintain its sterility. After fluid has filled the tubing, recap the end of the tubing.

11. If an electronic device is to be used, follow the manufacturer's instructions for inserting tubing into the device.

Initiate Peripheral Venous Access

12. Place the patient in low-Fowler's position in bed. Place protective towel or pad under patient's arm.

13. Provide emotional support, as needed.

14. Open the short extension tubing package. Attach the end cap, if not in place. Clean the end cap with an alcohol wipe. Insert the syringe with normal saline into the extension tubing. Fill the extension tubing with normal saline and apply the slide clamp. Remove the syringe and place the extension tubing and syringe back on the package, within easy reach.

15. Select and palpate for an appropriate vein. If the intended insertion site is visibly soiled, clean the area with soap and water.

16. If the site is hairy and agency policy permits, clip a 2-inch area around the intended entry site.

17. Put on gloves.

Excellent

Satisfactory

Needs Practice

SKILL 39-1

Initiating a Peripheral Venous Access
IV Infusion *(Continued)*

Comments

Excellent	Satisfactory	Needs Practice		Comments
——	——	——	18. Apply a tourniquet 3 to 4 inches above the venipuncture site to obstruct venous blood flow and distend the vein. Direct the ends of the tourniquet away from the entry site. Make sure the radial pulse is still present.	
——	——	——	19. Instruct the patient to hold the arm lower than the heart.	
——	——	——	20. Ask the patient to open and close the fist. Observe and palpate for a suitable vein. Try the following techniques if a vein cannot be felt:	
——	——	——	a. Lightly stroke the vein downward.	
——	——	——	b. Remove the tourniquet and place warm, dry compresses over the intended vein for 10 to 15 minutes.	
——	——	——	21. *Cleanse site with an antiseptic solution such as chlorhexidine or according to facility policy. Press the applicator against the skin and apply chlorhexidine, using a gentle back-and-forth motion. Do not wipe or blot. Allow to dry completely.*	
——	——	——	22. Alternately, for patients who bruise easily, are at risk for bleeding, or have fragile skin, *apply the chlorhexidine without scrubbing for at least 30 seconds. Allow to dry completely. Do not wipe or blot.*	
——	——	——	23. Using your nondominant hand placed about 1 or 2 inches below the entry site, hold the skin taut against the vein. *Avoid touching the prepared site.* Ask the patient to remain still while performing the venipuncture.	
——	——	——	24. Enter the skin gently, holding the catheter by the hub in your dominant hand, bevel side up, at a 10- to 15-degree angle. Insert the catheter from directly over the vein or from the side of the vein. While following the course of the vein, advance the needle or catheter into the vein. A sensation of "give" can be felt when the needle enters the vein.	
——	——	——	25. When blood returns through the lumen of the needle or the flashback chamber of the catheter, advance either device into the vein until the hub is at the venipuncture site. The exact technique depends on the type of device used.	
——	——	——	26. Release the tourniquet. Quickly remove the protective cap from the extension tubing and attach it to the catheter or needle. Stabilize the catheter or needle with your nondominant hand.	
——	——	——	27. Continue to stabilize the catheter or needle and flush gently with the saline, observing the site for infiltration and leaking.	

Excellent	Satisfactory	Needs Practice		Comments

28. Open the skin protectant wipe. Apply the skin protectant to the site, making sure to apply—at minimum—the area to be covered with the dressing. Place a sterile transparent dressing or catheter securing/stabilization device over the venipuncture site. Loop the tubing near the site of entry, and anchor with tape (nonallergenic) close to the site.

29. Label the IV dressing with the date, time, site, and type and size of catheter or needle used for the infusion.

30. Using an antimicrobial swab, cleanse the access cap on the extension tubing. Remove the end cap from the administration set. Insert the end of the administration set into the end cap. Loop the administration set tubing near the site of entry, and anchor with tape (nonallergenic) close to the site. Remove gloves.

31. Open the clamp on the administration set. Set the flow rate and begin the fluid infusion. Alternately, start the flow of solution by releasing the clamp on the tubing and counting the drops. Adjust until the correct drop rate is achieved. Assess the flow of the solution and function of the infusion device. Inspect the insertion site for signs of infiltration.

32. Apply an IV securement/stabilization device if not already in place as part of the dressing, as indicated, based on facility policy. Explain to the patient the purpose of the device and the importance of safeguarding the site when using the extremity.

33. Remove equipment and return the patient to a position of comfort. Lower the bed, if not in the lowest position.

34. Remove additional PPE, if used. Perform hand hygiene.

35. Return to check flow rate and observe IV site for infiltration and/or other complications 30 minutes after starting infusion, and at least hourly thereafter. Ask the patient if he or she is experiencing any pain or discomfort related to the IV infusion.

Skill Checklists for Fundamentals of Nursing: The Art and Science of Person-Centered Nursing Care, 8th edition

Name ______________________ Date ______________________

Unit ______________________ Position ______________________

Instructor/Evaluator: ______________________ Position ______________________

SKILL 39-2

Monitoring an IV Site and Infusion

Excellent	Satisfactory	Needs Practice	**Goal:** The patient remains free from complications and demonstrates signs and symptoms of fluid balance.	**Comments**
___	___	___	1. Verify the IV solution order on the MAR/CMAR with the medical order. Consider the appropriateness of the prescribed therapy in relation to the patient. Clarify any inconsistencies. Check the patient's chart for allergies. Check for color, leaking, and expiration date. Know the purpose of the IV administration and medications, if ordered.	
___	___	___	2. ***Monitor IV infusion every hour or per facility policy. More frequent checks may be necessary if medication is being infused.***	
___	___	___	3. Perform hand hygiene and put on PPE, if indicated.	
___	___	___	4. Identify the patient.	
___	___	___	5. Close the curtains around the bed and close the door to the room, if possible. Explain what you are going to do and why you are going to do it to the patient.	
___	___	___	6. If an electronic infusion device is being used, check settings, alarm, and indicator lights. Check set infusion rate. Note the position of the fluid in the IV container in relation to the time tape. Teach the patient about the alarm features on the electronic infusion device.	
___	___	___	7. If the IV is infusing via gravity, check the drip chamber and time the drops.	
___	___	___	8. Check the tubing for anything that might interfere with the flow. Be sure clamps are in the open position.	
___	___	___	9. Observe the dressing for leakage of IV solution.	
___	___	___	10. Inspect the site for swelling, leakage at the site, coolness, or pallor, which may indicate infiltration. Ask if the patient is experiencing any pain or discomfort. If any of these symptoms are present, the IV will need to be removed and restarted at another site. Check facility policy for treating infiltration.	

Excellent	Satisfactory	Needs Practice		Comments
— — —			11. Inspect the site for redness, swelling, and heat. Palpate for induration. Ask if the patient is experiencing pain. These findings may indicate phlebitis. Notify the primary care provider if phlebitis is suspected. The IV will need to be discontinued and restarted at another site. Check facility policy for treatment of phlebitis.	
— — —			12. Check for local manifestations (redness, pus, warmth, induration, and pain) that may indicate an infection is present at the site. Also check for systemic manifestations (chills, fever, tachycardia, hypotension) that may accompany local infection at the site. If signs of infection are present, discontinue the IV and notify the primary care provider. Be careful not to disconnect the IV tubing when putting on the patient's hospital gown or assisting the patient with movement.	
— — —			13. Be alert for additional complications of IV therapy, such as fluid overload bleeding.	
— — —			a. Fluid overload can result in signs of cardiac and/or respiratory failure. Monitor intake and output and vital signs. Assess for edema and auscultate lung sounds. Ask if the patient is experiencing any shortness of breath.	
— — —			b. Check for bleeding at the site.	
— — —			14. If appropriate, instruct the patient to call for assistance if any discomfort is noted at the site, the solution container is nearly empty, the flow has changed in any way, or if the electronic pump alarm sounds.	
— — —			15. Remove PPE, if used. Perform hand hygiene.	

Skill Checklists for Fundamentals of Nursing:
The Art and Science of Person-Centered Nursing Care, 8th edition

Name _____ Date _____

Unit _____ Position _____

Instructor/Evaluator: _____ Position _____

SKILL 39-3

Changing an IV Solution Container and Administration Set

Goal: The prescribed IV infusion continues without interruption and with infusion complications identified.

Excellent	Satisfactory	Needs Practice		Comments
——	——	——	1. Verify the IV solution order on the MAR/CMAR with the medical order. Consider the appropriateness of the prescribed therapy in relation to the patient. Clarify any inconsistencies. Check the patient's chart for allergies. Check for color, leaking, and expiration date. Know the purpose of the IV administration, and medications if ordered. Gather necessary supplies.	
——	——	——	2. Perform hand hygiene and put on PPE, if indicated.	
——	——	——	3. Identify the patient.	
——	——	——	4. Close the curtains around the bed and close the door to the room, if possible. Explain what you are going to do and why you are going to do it to the patient. Ask the patient about allergies to medications or tape, as appropriate.	
——	——	——	5. Compare the IV container label with the MAR/CMAR. Remove the IV bag from the outer wrapper, if indicated. Check expiration dates. Scan the bar code on the container, if necessary. Compare the patient identification band with the MAR/CMAR. Alternately, label the solution container with the patient's name, solution type, additives, date, and time. Complete a time strip for the infusion and apply to the IV container.	
——	——	——	6. Maintain aseptic technique when opening sterile packages and the IV solution. Remove the administration set from the package. Apply the label to the tubing, reflecting the day/date for next set change, per facility guidelines.	

To Change IV Solution Container

Excellent	Satisfactory	Needs Practice		Comments
——	——	——	7. If using an electronic infusion device, pause the device or put on "hold." Close the slide clamp on the administration set closest to the drip chamber. If using gravity infusion, close the roller clamp on the administration set.	
——	——	——	8. Carefully remove the cap on the entry site of the new IV solution container and expose the entry site, *taking care not to touch the exposed entry site.*	

Excellent	Satisfactory	Needs Practice	SKILL 39-3 **Changing an IV Solution Container and Administration Set** *(Continued)*	
				Comments
——	——	——	9. Lift the empty container off the IV pole and invert it. Quickly remove the spike from the old IV container, *being careful not to contaminate it.* Discard the old IV container.	
——	——	——	10. Using a twisting and pushing motion, insert the administration set spike into the entry site of the IV container. Alternately, follow the manufacturer's directions for insertion. Hang the container on the IV pole.	
——	——	——	11. Alternately, hang the new IV fluid container on an open hook on the IV pole. Carefully remove the cap on the entry site of the new IV solution container and expose the entry site, *taking care not to touch the exposed entry site.* Lift the empty container off the IV pole and invert it. Quickly remove the spike from the old IV container, *being careful not to contaminate it.* Discard the old IV container. Using a twisting and pushing motion, insert the administration set spike into the entry port of the new IV container as it hangs on the IV pole.	
——	——	——	12. If using an electronic infusion device, open the slide clamp, check the drip chamber of the administration set, verify the flow rate programmed in the infusion device, and turn the device to "run" or "infuse."	
——	——	——	13. If using gravity infusion, slowly open the roller clamp on the administration set and count the drops. Adjust until the correct drop rate is achieved.	
			To Change the IV Solution Container and Administration Set	
——	——	——	14. Prepare the IV solution and administration set.	
——	——	——	15. Hang the IV container on an open hook on the IV pole. Close the clamp on the existing IV administration set. Also, close the clamp on the short extension tubing connected to the IV catheter in the patient's arm.	
——	——	——	16. If using an electronic infusion device, remove the current administration set from the device. Following the manufacturer's directions, insert a new administration set into the infusion device.	
——	——	——	17. Put on gloves. Remove the current infusion tubing from the access cap on the short extension IV tubing. Using an antimicrobial swab, cleanse the access cap on the extension tubing. Remove the end cap from the new administration set. Insert the end of the administration set into the access cap. Loop the administration set tubing near the entry site, and anchor with tape (nonallergenic) close to the site.	

SKILL 39-3

Changing an IV Solution Container
and Administration Set *(Continued)*

Excellent	Satisfactory	Needs Practice		Comments
——	——	——	18. Open the clamp on the extension tubing. Open the clamp on the administration set.	
——	——	——	19. If using an electronic infusion device, open the slide clamp, check the drip chamber of the administration set, verify the flow rate programmed in the infusion device, and turn the device to "run" or "infuse."	
——	——	——	20. If using gravity infusion, slowly open the roller clamp on the administration set and count the drops. Adjust until the correct drop rate is achieved.	
——	——	——	21. Remove equipment. Ensure patient's comfort. Remove gloves. Lower the bed if not in the lowest position.	
——	——	——	22. Remove additional PPE, if used. Perform hand hygiene.	
——	——	——	23. Return to check the flow rate and observe the IV site for infiltration and/or other complications 30 minutes after starting infusion, and at least hourly thereafter. Ask if the patient is experiencing any pain or discomfort related to the IV infusion.	

Skill Checklists for Fundamentals of Nursing:
The Art and Science of Person-Centered Nursing Care, 8th edition

Name _____ Date _____

Unit _____ Position _____

Instructor/Evaluator: _____ Position _____

SKILL 39-4

Changing a Peripheral Venous Access Dressing

Goal: The patient exhibits an access site that is clean, dry, and without evidence of any signs and symptoms of infection, infiltration, or phlebitis. In addition, the dressing will be clean, dry, and intact and the patient will not experience injury.

Excellent	Satisfactory	Needs Practice		Comments
___	___	___	1. Determine the need for a dressing change. Check facility policy. Gather equipment.	
___	___	___	2. Perform hand hygiene and put on PPE, if indicated.	
___	___	___	3. Identify the patient.	
___	___	___	4. Close the curtains around the bed and close the door to the room, if possible. Explain what you are going to do and why you are going to do it to the patient. Ask the patient about allergies to tape and skin antiseptics.	
___	___	___	5. Put on gloves. Place a towel or disposable pad under the arm with the venous access. If solution is currently infusing, temporarily stop the infusion. Hold the catheter in place with your nondominant hand and *carefully remove old dressing and/or stabilization/securing device.* Use adhesive remover as necessary. Discard the dressing.	
___	___	___	6. *Inspect the IV site for presence of phlebitis (inflammation), infection, or infiltration.* Discontinue and relocate the IV, if noted.	
___	___	___	7. *Cleanse the site with an antiseptic solution such as chlorhexidine or according to facility policy. Press an applicator against the skin and apply chlorhexidine using a gentle back-and-forth motion. Do not wipe or blot. Allow to dry completely.*	
___	___	___	8. Open the skin protectant wipe. Apply the skin protectant to the site, making sure to cover at minimum the area to be covered with the dressing. Allow to dry. Place a sterile transparent dressing or catheter securing/stabilization device over the venipuncture site.	
___	___	___	9. Label the dressing with the date, time of change, and initials. Loop the tubing near the entry site and anchor with tape (nonallergenic) close to the site. Resume fluid infusion, if indicated. Check that IV flow is accurate and system is patent.	

Excellent	Satisfactory	Needs Practice		Comments

SKILL 39-4

Changing a Peripheral Venous
Access Dressing *(Continued)*

____ ____ ____ 10. Apply an IV securement/stabilization device if not already in place as part of the dressing, as indicated, based on facility policy. Explain to the patient the purpose of the device and the importance of safeguarding the site when using the extremity.

____ ____ ____ 11. Remove equipment. Ensure patient's comfort. Remove gloves. Lower the bed if not in the lowest position.

____ ____ ____ 12. Remove additional PPE, if used. Perform hand hygiene.

Skill Checklists for Fundamentals of Nursing:
The Art and Science of Person-Centered Nursing Care, 8th edition

Name _____ Date _____

Unit _____ Position _____

Instructor/Evaluator: _____ Position _____

SKILL 39-5

Capping for Intermittent Use and Flushing a Peripheral Venous Access Device

Goal: The patient remains free of injury and any signs and symptoms of IV complications.

Excellent	Satisfactory	Needs Practice		Comments
——	——	——	1. Determine the need for conversion to an intermittent access. Verify the medical order. Check facility policy. Gather equipment.	
——	——	——	2. Perform hand hygiene and put on PPE, if indicated.	
——	——	——	3. Identify the patient.	
——	——	——	4. Close the curtains around the bed and close the door to the room, if possible. Explain what you are going to do and why you are going to do it to the patient. Ask the patient about allergies to tape and skin antiseptics.	
——	——	——	5. Assess the IV site.	
——	——	——	6. If using an electronic infusion device, stop the device. Close the roller clamp on the administration set. If using gravity infusion, close the roller clamp on the administration set.	
——	——	——	7. Put on gloves. Close the clamp on the short extension tubing connected to the IV catheter in the patient's arm.	
——	——	——	8. Remove the administration set tubing from the extension set. Cleanse the end cap with an antimicrobial swab.	
——	——	——	9. Insert the saline flush syringe into the cap on the extension tubing. Pull back on the syringe to aspirate the catheter for positive blood return. If positive, instill the solution over 1 minute or flush the line according to facility policy. Remove the syringe and reclamp the extension tubing.	
——	——	——	10. If necessary, loop the extension tubing near the entry site and anchor it with tape (nonallergenic) close to the site.	
——	——	——	11. Remove equipment. Ensure patient's comfort. Remove gloves. Lower the bed if not in the lowest position.	
——	——	——	12. Remove additional PPE, if used. Perform hand hygiene.	

Name _____   Date _____

Unit _____   Position _____

Instructor/Evaluator: _____   Position _____

SKILL 39-6

Administering a Blood Transfusion

Excellent	Satisfactory	Needs Practice	**Goal:** The patient receives the blood transfusion without any evidence of a transfusion reaction or complication.	Comments
___	___	___	1. Verify the medical order for transfusion of a blood product. Verify the completion of informed consent documentation in the medical record. Verify any medical order for pretransfusion medication. If ordered, administer medication at least 30 minutes before initiating transfusion.	
___	___	___	2. Gather all equipment.	
___	___	___	3. Perform hand hygiene and put on PPE, if indicated.	
___	___	___	4. Identify the patient.	
___	___	___	5. Close the curtains around the bed and close the door to the room, if possible. Explain what you are going to do and why you are going to do it to the patient. Ask the patient about previous experience with transfusion and any reactions. Advise the patient to report any chills, itching, rash, or unusual symptoms.	
___	___	___	6. Prime the blood administration set with the normal saline IV fluid.	
___	___	___	7. Put on gloves. If patient does not have a venous access in place, initiate peripheral venous access. Connect the administration set to the venous access device via the extension tubing. Infuse the normal saline per facility policy.	
___	___	___	8. Obtain the blood product from the blood bank according to agency policy. Scan for bar codes on blood products if required.	
			9. Two nurses compare and validate the following information with the medical record, patient identification band, and the label of the blood product:	
___	___	___	• Medical order for transfusion of the blood product	
___	___	___	• Informed consent	
___	___	___	• Patient identification number	
___	___	___	• Patient name	
___	___	___	• Blood group and type	
___	___	___	• Expiration date	
___	___	___	• Inspection of blood product for clots, clumping, gas bubbles	

			SKILL 39-6

SKILL 39-6
Administering a Blood Transfusion *(Continued)*

Excellent	Satisfactory	Needs Practice		Comments
——	——	——	10. *Obtain a baseline set of vital signs before beginning transfusion.*	
——	——	——	11. Put on gloves. If using an electronic infusion device, put the device on "hold." Close the roller clamp closest to the drip chamber on the saline side of the administration set. Close the roller clamp on the administration set below the infusion device. Alternately, if using infusion via gravity, close the roller clamp on the administration set.	
——	——	——	12. Close the roller clamp closest to the drip chamber on the blood product side of the administration set. Remove the protective cap from the access port on the blood container. Remove the cap from the access spike on the administration set. Using a pushing and twisting motion, insert the spike into the access port on the blood container, taking care not to contaminate the spike. Hang the blood container on the IV pole. Open the roller clamp on the blood side of the administration set. Squeeze the drip chamber until the in-line filter is saturated. Remove gloves.	
——	——	——	13. *Start administration slowly (no more than 25 to 50 mL for the first 15 minutes). Stay with the patient for the first 5 to 15 minutes of transfusion.* Open the roller clamp on the administration set below the infusion device. Set the flow rate and begin the transfusion. Alternately, start the flow of solution by releasing the clamp on the tubing and counting the drops. Adjust until the correct drop rate is achieved. Assess the flow of the blood and function of the infusion device. Inspect the insertion site for signs of infiltration.	
——	——	——	14. Observe the patient for flushing, dyspnea, itching, hives or rash, or any unusual comments.	
——	——	——	15. After the observation period (5 to 15 minutes), increase the infusion rate to the calculated rate to complete the infusion within the prescribed time frame, no more than 4 hours.	
——	——	——	16. Reassess vital signs after 15 minutes. Obtain vital signs thereafter according to facility policy and nursing assessment.	
——	——	——	17. Maintain the prescribed flow rate as ordered or as deemed appropriate based on the patient's overall condition, keeping in mind the outer limits for safe administration. Ongoing monitoring is crucial throughout the duration of the blood transfusion for early identification of any adverse reactions.	

SKILL 39-6

Administering a Blood Transfusion *(Continued)*

Excellent	Satisfactory	Needs Practice		Comments

18. *During transfusion, assess frequently for transfusion reaction. Stop blood transfusion if you suspect a reaction. Quickly replace the blood tubing with a new administration set primed with normal saline for IV infusion. Initiate an infusion of normal saline for IV at an open rate, usually 40 mL/hour. Obtain vital signs. Notify the primary care provider and blood bank.*

19. When transfusion is complete, close the roller clamp on the blood side of the administration set and open the roller clamp on the normal saline side of the administration set. Initiate infusion of normal saline. When all of the blood has infused into the patient, clamp the administration set. Obtain vital signs. Put on gloves. Cap the access site or resume the previous IV infusion. Dispose of blood-transfusion equipment or return it to the blood bank, according to facility policy.

20. Remove equipment. Ensure the patient's comfort. Remove gloves. Lower the bed if not in the lowest position.

21. Remove additional PPE, if used. Perform hand hygiene.

22. Monitor and assess the patient for one hour after the transfusion for signs and symptoms of delayed transfusion reaction. Provide patient education about signs and symptoms of delayed transfusion reactions.